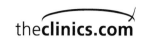
theclinics.com

OTOLARYNGOLOGIC CLINICS

OF NORTH AMERICA

Laryngeal Cancer

GUEST EDITORS
Nasir I. Bhatti, MD
Ralph P. Tufano, MD

August 2008 • Volume 41 • Number 4

SAUNDERS

An Imprint of Elsevier, Inc.
PHILADELPHIA   LONDON   TORONTO   MONTREAL   SYDNEY   TOKYO

W.B. SAUNDERS COMPANY
A Division of Elsevier Inc.

1600 John F. Kennedy Boulevard, Suite 1800, Philadelphia, PA 19103–2899

http://www.theclinics.com

OTOLARYNGOLOGIC CLINICS	Volume 41, Number 4
OF NORTH AMERICA	ISSN 0030–6665
August 2008	ISBN-13: 978-1-4160-5830-4
Editor: Joanne Husovski	ISBN-10: 1-4160-5830-3

Otolaryngologic Clinics of North America (ISSN 0030–6665) is published bimonthly by Elsevier Inc., 360 Park Avenue South, New York, NY 10010-1710. Months of issue are February, April, June, August, October, and December. Business and Editorial Offices: 1600 John F. Kennedy Blvd., Suite 1800, Philadelphia, PA 19103-2899. Customer Service Office: 6277 Sea Harbor Drive, Orlando, FL 32887-4800. Periodicals postage paid at New York, NY and additional mailing offices. Subscription price is $240.00 per year (US individuals), $448.00 per year (US institutions), $117.00 per year (US student/resident), $315.00 per year (Canadian individuals), $550.00 per year (Canadian institutions), $333.00 per year (international individuals), $550.00 per year (international institutions), $170.00 per year (international & Canadian student/resident). Foreign air speed delivery is included in all *Clinics'* subscription prices. All prices are subject to change without notice. **POSTMASTER:** Send address changes to *Otolaryngologic Clinics of North America*, Elsevier Periodicals Customer Service, 6277 Sea Harbor Drive, Orlando, FL 32887-4800. **Customer Service: 1-800-654-2452 (US). From outside the United States, call 1-407-563-6020. Fax: 1-407-563-8521. E-mail: JournalsCustomerService-usa@elsevier.com.**

Otolaryngologic Clinics of North America is also published in Spanish by McGraw-Hill Interamericana Editores S.A., P.O. Box 5-237, 06500 Mexico D.F., Mexico.

Otolaryngologic Clinics of North America is covered in *Index Medicus, Current Contents/Clinical Medicine, Excerpta Medica, BIOSIS, Science Citation Index,* and *ISI/BIOMED.*

Printed in the United States of America.

FOREWORD BY

CHARLES W. CUMMINGS, MD, Distinguished Service Professor, Otolaryngology, Head and Neck Surgery; Professor of Oncology, Johns Hopkins University School of Medicine, Baltimore, Maryland

GUEST EDITORS

NASIR I. BHATTI, MD, FACS, Associate Professor, Otolaryngology, Head and Neck Surgery, Johns Hopkins University School of Medicine, Baltimore, Maryland

RALPH P. TUFANO, MD, FACS, Associate Professor, Otolaryngology, Head and Neck Surgery, Johns Hopkins University School of Medicine, Baltimore, Maryland

CONTRIBUTORS

NISHANT AGRAWAL, MD, Department of Otolaryngology, Head and Neck Surgery, Johns Hopkins University School of Medicine, Baltimore, Maryland

NAFI AYGUN, MD, Assistant Professor of Radiology, Division of Neuroradiology, The Russell H. Morgan Department of Radiology and Radiological Science, Johns Hopkins University, Baltimore, Maryland

GOPAL K. BAJAJ, MD, Assistant Professor, Department of Radiation Oncology and Molecular Radiation Sciences, Johns Hopkins University School of Medicine, Baltimore, Maryland

ARI M. BLITZ, MD, Assistant Professor of Radiology, Division of Neuroradiology, The Russell H. Morgan Department of Radiology and Radiological Science, Johns Hopkins University, Baltimore, Maryland

EUGENE A. CHU, MD, Department of Otolaryngology, Head and Neck Surgery, Johns Hopkins University School of Medicine, Baltimore, Maryland

PAUL FLINT, MD, Professor, Department of Otolaryngology, Head and Neck Surgery, The Johns Hopkins University School of Medicine, Baltimore, Maryland

DAVID GOLDENBERG, MD, Associate Professor of Surgery, Director of Head and Neck Surgery, Department of Surgery, Division of Otolaryngology, Head and Neck Surgery, Pennsylvania State University College of Medicine, Hershey, Pennsylvania

PATRICK K. HA, MD, Assistant Professor, Department of Otolaryngology, Head and Neck Surgery, Johns Hopkins University School of Medicine; and The Milton J. Dance Center for Head and Neck Cancer, Greater Baltimore Medical Center, Baltimore, Maryland

ALEXANDER T. HILLEL, MD, Resident, Department of Otolaryngology, Head and Neck Surgery, Johns Hopkins University School of Medicine, Baltimore, Maryland

BORIS HRISTOV, MD, Resident Physician (PGY-3), Department of Radiation Oncology and Molecular Radiation Sciences, Johns Hopkins University School of Medicine, Baltimore, Maryland

ANKUR KAPOOR, PhD, Post-Doctoral Fellow, Department of Computer Science Whiting School of Engineering, The Johns Hopkins University, Baltimore, Maryland

YOUNG J. KIM, MD, PhD, Department of Otolaryngology, Head and Neck Surgery, Johns Hopkins University School of Medicine, Baltimore, Maryland

MYRIAM LOYO, MD, Department of Otolaryngology, Head and Neck Surgery, Johns Hopkins University School of Medicine, Baltimore, Maryland

SARA I. PAI, MD, PhD, Assistant Professor, Department of Otolaryngology, Head and Neck Surgery, Johns Hopkins University School of Medicine, Baltimore, Maryland

NABIL SIMAAN, PhD, Assistant Professor, Department of Mechanical Engineering Columbia University, New York, New York

EDWARD M. STAFFORD, MD, Instructor, Department of Otolaryngology, Head and Neck Surgery, Johns Hopkins Outpatient Center, Baltimore, Maryland

HEATHER M. STARMER, MA, CCC-SLP, Assistant, Department of Otolaryngology, Head and Neck Surgery, Johns Hopkins University, Baltimore, Maryland

RUSSELL H. TAYLOR, PhD, Professor, Department of Computer Science Whiting School of Engineering, Johns Hopkins University, Baltimore, Maryland

DONNA C. TIPPETT, MPH, MA, CCC-SLP, Assistant Professor, Department of Otolaryngology, Head and Neck Surgery, and Department of Physical Medicine and Rehabilitation, Johns Hopkins University, Baltimore, Maryland

RALPH P. TUFANO, MD, Associate Professor, Department of Otolaryngology, Head and Neck Surgery, Johns Hopkins Outpatient Center, Baltimore, Maryland

KIMBERLY T. WEBSTER, MA, MS, CCC-SLP, Johns Hopkins University, Baltimore, Maryland; and Assistant, Department of Otolaryngology, Head and Neck Surgery, Johns Hopkins Outpatient Center, Baltimore, Maryland

CONTENTS

there may be differences in cost and voice outcomes. Tumor factors, patient factors, and physician and patient preferences should dictate the choice of therapy.

FORTHCOMING ISSUES

RECENT ISSUES

The Clinics are now available online!

Access your subscription at
www.theclinics.com

ELSEVIER
SAUNDERS

Otolaryngol Clin N Am
41 (2008) ix–x

OTOLARYNGOLOGIC
CLINICS
OF NORTH AMERICA

Foreword

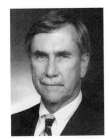

Charles W. Cummings, MD

I want to congratulate Drs. Bhatti and Tufano and their colleagues on this update of *Otolaryngologic Clinics of North America* involving "Management of Laryngeal Malignancy." This issue chronicles the continued evolution crafted by the talented core of Head and Neck Oncologists in our field. There is continued emphasis on the preservation of laryngeal function (or more specifically, restitution of laryngeal function) should it be compromised by disease or specific treatment. Please note that the parameters of laryngeal surgery are ever expansive, such that subtotal and extended, partial laryngectomies take on new dimensions three dimensionally.

Surgical techniques are in constant evolution, with the emphasis upon tissue sparing being paramount. New tools are being made available to the laryngeal surgical workforce, such as high frequency hemostatic cutting instrumentation, surgical debriders, tunable lasers—all playing a role. In addition, surgical access has been expanded by phenomenal fiber optic visualization, enhanced operative site illumination, flawless transfer from the operative site to the video screen, instrument miniaturization, and finally, the introduction of laryngeal robotic surgery which, coupled with the enhanced visualization, creates more precise surgical intervention.

Chemoradiation continues to provide a meaningful and oft-times attractive alternative to large-scale extirpative surgery. As the interval from the initial implementation of chemoradiation therapy lengthens, we are able to see more definitively some of the morbidity associated with this method of treatment. Disabling dysphasia looms as the most significant downside to the treatment, other than therapeutic failure.

doi:10.1016/j.otc.2008.01.022

It is apparent that progress is being accomplished, even though the steps are less grand than they once were. Still, I think that we will experience two giant steps in the not too distant future. The concept of tumor-specific tagged antibodies as a magic bullet is gaining a foothold in the treatment of lymphomas and other oncologic disorders. I am certain that this technology will fall to the realm of airway tumors and one can only imagine the potential for functional rehabilitation this methodology will offer. Similarly, the ability to provide a meaningful genetic assay will allow us to identify those who are at risk for airway tumors and allow us to be more proactive with respect to diagnosis and subsequent definitive treatment.

I am confident that the great strides being made in the basic science laboratories, coupled with the systematic translation of new technology to the bedside, augers well for meaningful advances in the quest to achieve conquest over laryngeal oncologic disease.

Charles W. Cummings, MD
Distinguished Service Professor
Otolaryngology Head and Neck Surgery
Professor of Oncology
Johns Hopkins University School of Medicine
601 N. Caroline Street
Baltimore, MD 21287, USA

ELSEVIER
SAUNDERS

Otolaryngol Clin N Am
41 (2008) xi–xii

OTOLARYNGOLOGIC
CLINICS
OF NORTH AMERICA

Preface

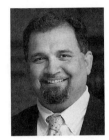 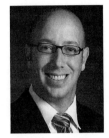

Nasir I. Bhatti, MD, FACS   Ralph P. Tufano, MD, FACS
Guest Editors

There has been speculation by some that the aspect of medicine as an art form no longer exists. Nowhere is that more incorrect than in dealing with laryngeal malignancies. The multidisciplinary care rendered from diagnosis to rehabilitation requires creative problem solving because each patient is so different. Successful oncologic and functional outcomes are dependent on the creativity and careful thought processes of the multidisciplinary team. The role of multidisciplinary tumor conferences can not be overemphasized. Surgical options now run the gamut, from minimally invasive endoscopic procedures to technically challenging open procedures with predictable outcomes.

Advances in chemotherapeutic agents, radiation therapy modalities, and imaging technologies have expanded our armamentarium to fight this disease. There has been an appreciation of the complex interplay of psychosocial and physical factors that have helped plan optimal, individually tailored rehabilitation strategies. The future promises robotic surgery advances to help more precisely define tumor resection and spare function. Molecular biology advances are forthcoming, which will allow us to profile tumor behavior and design even more tailored treatment protocols.

This issue of *Otolaryngologic Clinics of North America* addresses these dynamic aspects of laryngeal cancer management, and provides an overview of the complex considerations one must appreciate when managing laryngeal cancer to maximize oncologic and functional outcomes for our patients. We are deeply indebted to our colleagues for providing the readership with the current state-of-the-art knowledge and concepts in this regard.

This issue is dedicated to our parents, family, mentors, and all who aspire to provide the most comprehensive and state-of-the-art management of laryngeal cancer.

Nasir I. Bhatti, MD, FACS
Associate Professor
Otolaryngology Head and Neck Surgery
Johns Hopkins University School of Medicine
Room 6241, 601 North Caroline Street
Baltimore, MD 21287, USA

E-mail address: nbahatti@jhmi.edu

Ralph P. Tufano, MD, FACS
Associate Professor
Otolaryngology Head and Neck Surgery
Johns Hopkins University School of Medicine
601 North Caroline Street, 6th floor
Baltimore, MD 21287-0910, USA

E-mail address: rtufano@jhmi.edu

OTOLARYNGOLOGIC
CLINICS
OF NORTH AMERICA

Otolaryngol Clin N Am
41 (2008) 657–672

ELSEVIER
SAUNDERS

The Molecular Genetics
of Laryngeal Cancer

Myriam Loyo, MD, Sara I. Pai, MD, PhD*

*Department of Otolaryngology, Head and Neck Surgery, Johns Hopkins University School
of Medicine, 601 North Caroline Street, Baltimore, MD 21287, USA*

The incidence of laryngeal cancer in the United States was estimated to be 11,300 in 2007 [1]. Although the quality of life of patients who have laryngeal cancer has improved with organ preservation approaches in recent years, the survival rate for laryngeal cancer has remained unchanged in the past 30 years [2]. At the time of diagnosis, approximately 42% of patients have disease localized to the primary site, 47% have lymph node metastasis, and 7% have distant metastasis [1]. Patients who have laryngeal cancer are at risk for developing second primary tumors at a rate of 14% at 5 years, 26% at 10 years, and 37% at 15 years [3]. These high rates of second primary tumor development may be attributed to the field cancerization effect. Recent discoveries in the molecular biology of head and neck squamous cell carcinoma (HNSCC), and of laryngeal carcinoma in particular, can provide insight to understanding the molecular basis of these cancers, which can lead to the development of early diagnostic and targeted therapeutic strategies aimed to improve clinical outcomes, and possibly survival, in this patient population.

Causative risk factors

Tobacco use and alcohol consumption are well-established risk factors for HNSCC. The larynx has been suggested to be the organ most susceptible to carcinogenic insult from tobacco smoke in the head and neck region [4]. The enzymes that metabolize the carcinogenic compounds in cigarettes and alcohol, such as glutathione S-transferase, N-acetyltransferase, cytochrome p450, alcohol dehydrogenase, and aldehyde dehydrogenase, have been studied to assess an individual's risk for cancer development, and although

* Corresponding author. 601 North Caroline Street, Baltimore, MD 21287.
E-mail address: spai@jhmi.edu (S.I. Pai).

considerable polymorphisms of these enzymes have been found among the population, the results are controversial [2,5,6]. Although tobacco exposure and alcohol consumption are the etiologic causes for approximately 75% to 80% of HNSCC, infection with the human papillomavirus (HPV) has been etiologically linked with the remaining 20% to 25% of all head and neck cancers [7–9]. Upon infection of the cell, the HPV E6 and E7 viral proteins bind and disrupt two important cellular gatekeeper proteins, *p53* and *pRb*, respectively [10]. In laryngeal cancer, the prevalence of HPV DNA has been reported to range between 3% and 47% [11]. The wide variation in prevalence is most likely attributable to the various detection techniques used. In addition to detection of the "high-risk" HPV types, such as HPV-16 and HPV-18, which are associated with oropharyngeal cancers, there are several studies that have reported the integration of the HPV-11 genome in patients who have recurrent respiratory papillomatosis and who progressed to develop carcinoma [12–14]. However, further studies are necessary before a clear association between HPV and laryngeal cancer can be established.

Genetic progression model

In 1971, Knudson proposed that loss of both parental alleles of a tumor suppressor gene (TSG) can lead to a malignant phenotype [15]. In 1990, Fearon and Vogelstein [16] expanded this concept and proposed that either loss of TSGs and/or activation of oncogenes can lead to cellular transformation, and it is the progressive accumulation of such genetic alterations which can lead to a selective growth advantage of a clonal population of transformed cells which can then develop into cancer. Statistical analysis based on the age-specific incidence of head and neck cancer suggests that HNSCCs arise after the accumulation of 6-10 independent genetic events. Taking these concepts, a progression model can be established by tracking the genetic changes acquired through time within cloneal populations and then correlating these genetic changes with histologic progression from hyperplasia, to dysplasia, to carcinoma in situ, and, finally, to invasive carcinoma. The techniques that can be used to track the molecular alterations include cytogenetics, loss of heterozygosity (LOH), mutation analysis, and, more recently, gene expression profiles.

Cytogenetics is the analysis of chromosomes for structural changes, such as translocations, deletions, or amplifications. The classic karyotype and fluorescence in situ hybridization (FISH) assays are commonly used cytogenetic techniques. The former uses trypsin-Giemsa staining to compare the banding of the chromosomes, and the latter localizes particular regions of the chromosome with DNA probes. Since the size of the alterations needs to be large enough to be visualized on a microscopic scale, these tests are considered to have low sensitivity.

A more sensitive test is the detection of specific allelic loss or LOH. The assay consists of a polymerase chain reaction (PCR) that amplifies microsatellite markers, which are short repeat polymorphic regions distributed throughout the noncoding genome. The loss of microsatellite markers in the assay identifies areas of neighboring alleles harboring potential TSGs, and the implication of the functional deficit of the protein is the development of carcinogenesis. This technique evaluates gene expression or deletion within a localized region of the chromosome. With the advent of microarray technology, whole genome gene expression profiling is now possible. Comparison of gene expression patterns between normal and cancerous cells enables the characterization of gene expression patterns that can be correlated with functionally important genes or states. For example, using microarray technology, tumor classifications, treatment responses, and clinical outcome predictions may become a reality in many cancers. This area of research is actively evolving with the generation of novel assays that provide reliable, sensitive, high-throughput assays with accurate and efficient read-out systems of thousands of genes.

In 1996, Califano and colleagues [17] correlated histologic progression from hyperplasia, to dysplasia, to carcinoma in situ, and to invasive carcinoma by tracking genetic changes acquired through time using LOH and FISH analysis and proposed a genetic progression model for head and neck cancer. The group found that 30% of head and neck precursor cancer lesions, such as hyperplasia, showed loss of chromosome 9p21, indicating that loss in this region was an early event. This locus was found to encode *p16* (CDKN2A/MTS1), an important TSG that inhibits cell cycle progression from the G1 checkpoint to the S phase by inhibiting the phosphorylation of p*Rb*. Dyplasia demonstrated genetic alterations with loss of 3p21 and 17p13. The latter locus contains *p53*, which is a major TSG that plays an important regulatory role in DNA repair, cell cycle progression, and apoptosis. Carcinoma in situ had loss of 13q21 and 14q32 and amplification of 11q3. p*Rb* is contained in the 13q21 region and controls cell cycle progression *Cyclin D* (PRAD1) is localized to the 11q3 locus and overexpression of this gene results in phosphorylation, and thus activation of p*Rb*. Invasive carcinomas were found to have LOH on 6p, 8p, 4p27, and 10q12 [16]. Subsequent multiple studies have confirmed chromosomal losses on 3p, 5q, 8p, 9p, 13p, 18q, and 21q in head and neck cancers [17–20].

The establishment of a genetic progression model has several advantages. The use of allelic loss may facilitate the prediction of the malignant potential of low-grade premalignant lesions. It has been found that patients with 3p and 9p loss have a 3.8-fold risk for progression to cancer. Additional losses, such as 4q, 8p, 11q, or 17p, increase the risk to 33-fold, however [21,22]. Therefore, patients with LOH at 3p or 9p are at risk for progression, and their relative risk increases with loss of additional arms. This information can be used to tailor treatment to the individual and his or her lesion. For example, patients with LOH at 3p or 9p with additional loss on other chromosomal arms may need more aggressive treatment of their lesions, whereas, patients with only 3p or 9p LOH may benefit from close monitoring for further alterations.

A genetic progression model can also guide the development of novel treatment strategies through gene therapy and the replacement of altered genes with their wild-type phenotype. Laryngeal cancer has a particular pattern of p53 mutations as compared with other regions of the head and neck. The laryngeal pattern is more consistent with that of lung cancer, and it shows lower mutation indexes (35.4% versus 60%) with different concentrated regions of *p53* mutations. In most head and neck cancers, exons 5 through 8 are altered, whereas in laryngeal cancer, the mutations tend to cluster in exon 5, especially in the S2 protein domain and in codon 248 [23]. A therapeutic strategy that is currently in development is the delivery of wild-type p53 into dysplastic or cancerous cells to restore wild-type p53 function within the cell. This approach has been explored using a recombinant adenovirus that delivers wild-type p53 (Ad5CMV-p53) in a laryngeal cancer model. In vivo studies demonstrated that intratumoral injections of Ad5CMV-p53 significantly inhibited the further growth of established laryngeal tumor xenografts [24]. Furthermore, studies have demonstrated that the cotransfer of wild-type p53 with immunomodulatory genes, such as granulocyte-macrophage colony-stimulating factor (GM-CSF) and B7-1 genes using a recombinant adenovirus, induced cellular apoptosis and enhanced the immunogenicity of cancer cells, suggesting a potential combinatorial gene therapy strategy for laryngeal cancer [25,26].

Epigenetic alterations

Genetic loss of function mutations, such as point mutations, deletions, and translocations, was one of the first identified means of silencing TSGs; however, it has been found that gene silencing can also be achieved by epigenetic alterations of the genome, such as DNA hypermethylation of CpG islands in the promoter regions of TSGs. DNA hypermethylation of a promoter region results in transcriptional suppression of the gene through the recruitment of chromatin remodeling complexes. Different epigenetic profiles have been found when comparing tumor with normal tissue, which has provided insight into genetic oncogenesis.

The main mechanisms for epigenetic silencing are DNA hypermethylation and chromatin modification. DNA hypermethylation refers to the addition of a methyl group to the cytosine ring from a methyl donor by a DNA methyltransferase (DNMT). This occurs in regions of the DNA in which there are high concentrations of cytosines followed by guanosines or CpG dinucleotides. These regions are called CpG islands and are present in the noncoding promoter regions. Detection assays for methylation can be targeted to specific genes or global genomes. Among the targeted techniques, a methylation-specific restriction enzyme assay with Southern blot analysis was the first to be used. Currently, PCR techniques are used after sodium bisulfite treatment, which converts nonmethylated cytosines into uracil and makes methylation detectable by the presence or absence of a PCR product on an agarose gel.

The p16 gene which is located on chromosome 9p21 is a region that has been found to be silenced through promoter hypermethylation. Genomic analysis of the p16 locus demonstrated that 67% of patients had a homozygous deletion of the p16 locus and 21% had hypermethylation of the p16 promoter [27]. In another study of 14 HNSCC cell lines, 21% of the lines had homozygous deletions of the locus, 29% had exonic mutations, 14% had intronic mutations, and 29% showed hypermethylation of the p16 promoter [27]. Investigations of other genes known to exhibit promoter hypermethylation in other cancers have revealed similar promoter hypermethylation patterns in HNSCC as well. For example, E-cadherin (CDH1) is involved in cell-to-cell adhesion and is methylated in 0% to 85% of HNSCC, O6-methylguanine-DNA methyltransferase (MGMT) plays a role in detoxifying DNA adducts and is methylated in 25% to 52% of HNSCC, and death-associated protein kinase (DAPK) is involved in apoptosis and is methylated in 7% to 68% of HNSCC [28–32]. The wide range of variation might be attributed to the different detection techniques used. The current challenge in epigenetics is identifying genes that are relevant and uniquely involved in HNSCC.

The methylation pattern of tumors has been evaluated within the tumor bed and in body fluids, such as serum or exfoliated cells shed by the tumor. A study involving 33 patients diagnosed with early stage laryngeal cancer detected p16 methylation in 42% of the pharyngoesophageal collections; combining it with UT5085 tetranucleotide microsatellite instability, this combination of genetic and epigenetic alterations were found in 76% of the tumors [33]. This study highlights the importance of combining genetic and epigenetic alterations when evaluating molecular changes in any cancer, because the combination of alterations may provide a better "fingerprint" of the cancer biology than any single approach.

Despite regional promoter hypermethylation, global hypomethylation is also present in HNSCC and other solid tumors. In a study looking at 134 samples, the global methylation level for HNSCC specimens was 46.8% and the methylation level for normal controls was 54% ($P < .001$). Hypomethylation levels were found to increase with tumor stage and in patients exposed to alcohol and tobacco smoke [34]. The implication of global hypomethylation is the potential reactivation of proto-oncogenes in contrast to hypermethylation, which is the silencing of TSGs. Epigenetic alterations are an interesting phenomenon, and as more insight is gained into this area of research, it should be interesting to see how epigenetic changes can be integrated into a head and neck tumor progression model.

Altered protein expression

In addition to genetic and epigenetic modifications, protein-based alterations may contribute to carcinogenesis. The epidermal growth factor receptor (EGFR; also known as HER1 and ErbB1) is a transmembrane tyrosine kinase (TK) receptor that plays a critical role in cell survival and proliferation. Activation of EGFR through ligand binding with the epidermal growth factor (EGF) or transforming growth factor-α (TGFα) leads to receptor dimerization, kinase activation, and autophosphorylation, which activate various cellular pathways involved in cellular proliferation, angiogenesis, metastases, and inhibition of apoptosis. More than 90% of HNSCC overexpresses EGFR [35–37]. In HPV-associated head and neck cancers, the viral protein E5 upregulates the expression of EGFR [9,38]; however, in non–HPV-associated HNSCC, the mechanisms for upregulation are not fully understood with gene amplification of the EGFR gene occuring in a low percentage of HNSCC (0%–25%) [39,40]. Therefore, alternative proposed mechanisms for overexpression include mutational activation of EGFR [41], overexpression of EGFR ligands, establishment of autocrine or paracrine loops [39,40], and transactivation by other receptor and nonreceptor TKs [35,36].

EGFR overexpression has been associated with an unfavorable prognosis in early glottic carcinomas [42] and has been linked to early disease progression, poor survival, and resistance to chemotherapy [9,38]. Therefore, blocking the EGFR signal transduction pathway has been evaluated as a potential target for anticancer therapy. The EGFR pathway can be targeted by monoclonal antibodies (mAbs) and by tyrosine kinase inhibitors (TKIs). Anti-EGFR antibodies, such as cetuximab, which is a chimerized mAb, act as competitive antagonists to the receptor ligands, such as EGF and TGFα. Suggested mechanisms of action of anti-EGFR mAb-based therapy include inhibition of ligand-induced activation of this receptor and induction of receptor degradation. Other potential mechanisms of therapy are antibody-dependent cellular cytotoxicity, complement-dependent cytotoxicity, and complement-dependent cell-mediated cytotoxicity [39,40,43]. In early clinical studies, single-agent activity of cetuximab was shown to be effective and safe in HNSCC [44–46]. The most common side effect was a skin rash, and less common side effects included fatigue, nausea, vomiting, diarrhea, mucositis, and hypersensitivity reactions. In a phase III randomized clinical trial that compared radiation therapy (RT) and cetuximab with RT alone, patients who had locally advanced HNSCC demonstrated better survival and locoregional control by 10% to 15%. Laryngeal preservation rates were also improved [47]. Consequently, in February 2006, the US Food and Drug Administration (FDA) approved cetuximab in combination with RT as a frontline treatment for patients who have locally advanced HNSCC [46,48–50]. Additional trials have been undertaken to assess the feasibility of combining cetuximab with chemo-RT. A phase II trial demonstrated that the combination of cetuximab with RT and cisplatin yielded 3-year overall survival, progression-free survival, and locoregional control rates of 76%, 56%, and 71%, respectively [51]. In addition, the combination of cetuximab with RT and gemcitabine in HNSCC yielded a complete response rate of 77%, with 89% patient compliance to chemotherapy [52].

In light of these promising results, several groups have addressed the potential benefit of inhibiting the EGFR pathway downstream of the extracellular EGFR domain by using other molecules, such as TKIs, that target the EGFR intracellular machinery. TKIs are small molecules that cross the plasma membrane and interact with the cytoplasmic domain of cell-surface receptors, which modulate intracellular signaling. They are less specific than mAbs and may be associated with increased toxicities because of the associated inhibition of several signaling pathways. Similar to the results obtained with single-agent mAbs, modest responses ranging between 1% and 11% were obtained with single-agent TKIs in phase II trials using gefitinib or erlotinib in patients who had recurrent or metastatic HNSCC. The combination of TKIs with chemotherapy or RT resulted in more favorable results, however [53]. A phase I/II trial of erlotinib and cisplatin in patients who had recurrent or metastatic HNSCC demonstrated a favorable toxicity profile and antitumor activity comparable to standard combination chemotherapy regimens [54].

Several recent reports suggest that dual-agent targeting of the EGFR pathway may overcome the limitations of a single agent to suppress EGFR-mediated signaling sufficiently. In a human tumor xenograft model, the combined treatment of gefitinib and cetuximab resulted in a synergistic effect on inhibiting cell proliferation [55]. A phase I study demonstrated that cetuximab combined with gefitinib enhanced tumor cell apoptosis and reduced proliferation rates of tumors as compared with a single agent alone in patients who had HNSCC [56].

As clinical trials that target the EGFR pathway continue to grow, the mechanisms underlying tumor resistance to or lack of sensitization by EGFR inhibitors will need to be addressed. One hypothesis for resistance to EGFR inhibitors is the presence of EGFR mutations in the extracellular domain, which results in a lack of recognition by mAbs, and in the intracellular domain, which results in a diminished response to EGFR antagonists. There are only a few somatic mutations of the EGFR gene reported in patients who had HNSCC, however. In Asian patients, the incidence rate was reported to be 7.3% (3 of 65 patients) [57]; in European patients, it was 1% (1 of 100 patients) [58]; and in American patients, no mutation has yet been detectable (0 of 65 patients) [57]. Other possible explanations for the limited efficacy of EGFR-directed therapy are the constitutive activation of signaling pathways downstream of EGFR or activation of EGFR-independent pathways, such as G protein–coupled receptors (GPCRs) [41], which may promote survival and resistance to EGFR inhibitors. Because of the potential of developing resistance to directed therapies, multimodality treatments that target multiple aberrant cellular pathways may be the appropriate strategy to improve overall clinical outcomes.

Alterations in tumor environment

The development and progression of cancer depend initially on genetic, epigenetic, and protein-based alterations within the clonal population; however, the cancer cells must then alter the microenvironment to support their continued growth. Matrix metalloproteinases (MMPs) are a family of proteolytic zinc-containing enzymes that are responsible for the breakdown of the extracellular matrix components. They are involved in basement membrane disruption, stroma and blood vessel penetration, and metastases [59,60]. Overexpression of MMP-9 has been observed in various tumors, including laryngeal lesions [55,56,61,62]. The expression levels of MMP-9 in 154 laryngeal lesions, including keratosis, papillomas, dysplasia, in situ carcinoma, and squamous cell carcinoma (SCC), were evaluated by immunohistochemistry [63]. Overexpression of MMP-9 was observed in 74.4% and 50% of invasive and in situ SCC, respectively. In dysplastic lesions papillomas, and keratoses, MMP-9 overexpression was 62.9%, 61.5%, and 54.2%, respectively. The overexpression of MMP-9 was statistically higher in invasive SCC as compared with dysplasias ($P < .05$). Therefore, it was concluded that the overexpression of MMP occurs in a stepwise fashion in the progression model, with the highest levels of overexpression occurring in invasive lesions [41,64]. Interestingly, the presence of MMP in the primary tumor has been investigated as a clinical surrogate marker for the prediction of nodal and distal metastasis and for the possibility of recurrence [9,38]. In a retrospective study of 72 patients who had laryngeal SCC, a significantly lower survival rate was found in patients with MMP-2 expression within their tumors ($P = .0028$), and its overexpression was indicative of increased risk for primary recurrence [65,66].

Angiogenesis also plays a central role in the pathogenesis of cancer. Angiogenic vessel formation is crucial to support tumor growth as the tumor demands for oxygen and nutrients increase. Vascular endothelial growth factor (VEGF) plays a fundamental role in tumor angiogenesis. In 2000, Smith and colleagues [67] reported VEGF expression as an independent risk factor for poor local-regional control and overall survival in HNSCC. A recent meta-analysis of patients who had HNSCC by Kyzas and colleagues [68] revealed that the risk for death in 2 years was almost two times higher in VEGF-expressing patients. In another retrospective study involving 76 patients who had laryngopharyngeal carcinoma, the expression levels of VEGF were associated with a 16.2-fold higher probability of cervical lymph node relapse ($P = .032$) and with an 8.44-fold shorter disease-free survival ($P = .045$), suggesting that VEGF expression is a predictive factor of cervical lymph node recurrence [69,70].

Because VEGF expression is associated with increased angiogenesis, tumor growth, and risk for recurrence, several VEGF and VEGFR antagonists have been developed. One such therapy is the recombinant humanized anti-VEGF mAb, bevacizumab, which neutralizes VEGF and blocks signal transduction. Bevacizumab has been shown to inhibit tumor growth significantly as a single-agent therapy in colorectal, renal cell, and non–small-cell lung cancers with observed synergistic effects when combined with chemotherapy or RT. Other approaches to reduce VEGF levels that are being explored are VEGF antisense oligonucleotides, RNA interference, and recombinant adenoviral vectors encoding a secreted form of the extracellular domain of VEGFR [71,72]. This is an exciting area of investigational research, and as our understanding of how the tumor is able to modulate its microenvironment advances, we can develop targeted therapies to counteract those changes that support tumor invasion and metastasis.

Immune evasion

In addition to modifying the local microenvironment to support their growth, tumors can alter the systemic environment to evade immune recognition or surveillance. Alterations in the immune functions of patients who have HNSCC have been documented. One of the first indications that the immune system was abnormal in patients who had HNSCC was the observation that patients lacked a delayed type hypersensitivity (DTH) reaction as compared with the normal adult population [73,74]. Since this initial observation, the mechanisms by which tumors escape immune surveillance have been extensively studied and continue to become elucidated. Several of the molecular strategies used by HNSCC to evade the immune system include the expression of immune suppressive mediators, altered tumor antigen processing and presentation, and impaired dendritic cell (DC) and lymphocyte function.

Studies of primary cultures of human HNSCC cells revealed high secretion levels of numerous immunosuppressive cytokines, such as interleukin (IL)-4, IL-6, IL-8, IL-10, and prostaglandin E_2 (PGE_2) [75]. In addition, it has been found that patients who have HNSCC have a bias toward the secretion of T helper 2 (TH_2), cytokines that prevent effective antitumor TH_1 immune responses against the tumor.

Defects in antigen-presenting cells, such as DCs, have also been described in patients who have HNSCC. In a study of 44 patients who had HNSCC, the capability of DCs generated from peripheral blood monocytes to form cell clusters with allogeneic lymphocytes was reduced compared with healthy controls [76]. The DC clustering capability was restored after surgical removal of the tumor [59,60], indicating a role of tumor-derived factors in the functional impairments of DCs in patients who have HNSCC. Functional impairments of monocyte and macrophage functions have also been documented in patients who have HNSCC. Decreased expression of D-related human leukocyte antigen (HLA-DR) by monocytes has been found, which results in decreased antigen presentation, and thus inactivation of cytoxic T cells [61,62]. One group reported that in 19 of 39 patients who had HNSCC, isolated macrophages were noncytotoxic toward the tumor cells and that 12 of 30 patients possessed a plasma inhibitory factor capable of suppressing macrophage-mediated cytotoxicity by more than 50% [77,78].

Other reported immunomodulatory molecules expressed by patients who have HNSCC are p15E-like and Fas ligand (FasL). The p15E-like factors have a high homology with the immunosuppressive retroviral protein p15E. The functional properties of p15E-like factors include suppression of peripheral mononuclear cell chemotaxis; inhibition of DC clustering; and suppression of monocyte-mediated killing, natural killer (NK)–cell activity, and B-cell activation [79,80].

In addition to suppressing immunologic cell function of antigen-presenting cells, tumors may alter cytotoxic T-cell function. Fas (Apo-1/CD95) is involved in the apoptotic pathway by activating caspase-3. The expression of Fas depends on tumor differentiation: it is more prominent in well-differentiated carcinomas, less prominent in moderately differentiated carcinomas, and absent in undifferentiated carcinomas (and in normal epithelium) [63,81]. The FasL can be shed by the tumor to induce apoptosis of Fas-expressing lymphocytes in patients who have HNSCC [82]. In addition to inducing apoptosis of tumor-infiltrating lymphocytes, recent studies have focused on functional T-cell impairments. Peripheral blood lymphocytes of healthy individuals proliferate when stimulated with phytohemagglutinin A in vitro; however, this response is decreased in patients who have HNSCC, and the severity of this impairment is correlated to tumor stage [67–70]. In addition, tumor-infiltrating lymphocytes isolated from HNSCC were found to have poor cytolytic function immediately after isolation; however, after in vitro culture of the cells in the presence of IL-2, these cells were capable of eliminating tumor cells [71–74], again suggesting the presence of tumor-derived inhibitory factors that dampen the immune response.

Because the immune system plays a critical role in the early detection and eradication of tumor cells, several different immunotherapy strategies have been evaluated for HNSCC. Biologic response modifiers, such as the introduction of ILs, represent a growing field. Encouraging results with systemic and local delivery of IL-2 in melanoma and renal cell carcinoma have prompted studies in HNSCC [83,84]. Using a murine orthotopic model of HNSCC, it was found that the combination of IL-2 delivery and external beam radiation generated potent antitumor immune responses with associated apoptosis of the tumor cells [85]. Furthermore, the addition of IL-12 to the combined treatment of IL-2 and external beam RT resulted in synergistic antitumor effects with increased tumor cell apoptosis and T-lymphocyte infiltration of CD4+ and CD8+ T cells in an orthotopic murine HNSCC model [82].

Other investigational immunomodulatory agents include the thymic hormone extract, thymostimulin (TP1), which has been shown to restore impaired monocyte chemotaxis and impaired capability of DCs to form cellular clusters, as often observed in patients who have HNSCC [86]. Sizofilan, a β-D-glucan obtained from the apyllophoral fungus *Schizophyllum commune Feries*, has been used as an immunoadjuvant and has been found to aid in the recovery of cellular immunity in patients who have cancer [87]. OK-432 is a lyophilized preparation of a low-virulence strain of

Streptococcus pyogenes that has been proposed as a noncytotoxic antineo-plastic agent because of its immune stimulating activity. The local injection of OK-432 attracts inflammatory cells to the lesion and correlates with a better clinical response through activation of the innate immune system [88]. Cancer vaccines are another strategy of enhancing the immune response in patients with HNSCC that is currently being explored. The identification of tumor-associated antigens that are uniquely expressed by the tumor facilitates the development of targeted cancer vaccines. The HPV E6 and E7 viral proteins are highly immunogenic and are currently being explored in clinical trials in patients who have HNSCC [89]. An approach gaining increasing popularity in the tumor vaccine field is to immunize patients who have cancer with autologous DCs loaded ex vivo with tumor antigens. The underlying premise of this approach is that ex vivo manipulation of the DCs is an efficient and controlled manner in which to generate synchronously activated DCs that provides a superior method for stimulating antitumor immunity in vivo compared with the more conventional direct vaccination methods.

Summary

A better understanding of the steps involved in malignant transformation can help to develop novel diagnostic, prognostic, and therapeutic strategies. Molecular diagnostics can detect abnormalities in lesions not yet appreciated histologically and may help in the detection of minimal residual disease or early recurrences. Specific molecular patterns can establish a tumor's behavior and help to guide patient management. Patients who have less aggressive tumors may safely undergo treatment with organ preservation, whereas patients who have more aggressive tumors may benefit from extended surgical or chemoradiation approaches. With a better understanding of the molecular genetics and epigenetics of laryngeal cancer, novel targeted therapies for HNSCC can be translated into the clinical arena. Several clinical trials are exploring the use of p53-engineered recombinant adenoviruses to restore wild-type gene function and the use of EGFR pathway antagonists. In addition, novel therapies directed at modifying the tumor microenvironment and immunologic responses directed against the cancer cell continue to pave the way for treatment options tailored to the individual patient and his or her cancer. As the molecular biology field continues to advance with gene expression profiling techniques, we hope to identify unique gene expression fingerprints of head and neck cancers that may help to classify tumors based on predicted clinical behavior, evaluate treatment responses, and direct therapies to improve clinical outcomes.

References

[1] Ries LAG, Melbert D, Krapcho M, et al, editors. SEER cancer statistics review, 1975–2004. Bethesda (MD): National Cancer Institute. Available at: http://seer.cancer.gov/csr/

1975_2004/. based on November 2006 SEER data submission, posted to the SEER web site, 2007.

[2] Almadori G, Bussu F, Cadoni G, et al. Molecular markers in laryngeal squamous cell carcinoma: towards an integrated clinicobiological approach. Eur J Cancer 2005;41:683–93.

[3] Gao X, Fisher SG, Mohideen N, et al. Second primary cancers in patients with laryngeal cancer: a population-based study. Int J Radiat Oncol Biol Phys 2003;56:427–35.

[4] Hashibe M, Brennan P, Benhamou S, et al. Alcohol drinking in never users of tobacco, cigarette smoking in never drinkers, and the risk of head and neck cancer: pooled analysis in the International Head and Neck Cancer Epidemiology Consortium. J Natl Cancer Inst 2007;99:777–89.

[5] Ha PK, Califano JA III. The molecular biology of laryngeal cancer. Otolaryngol Clin North Am 2002;35:993–1012.

[6] Ho T, Wei Q, Sturgis EM. Epidemiology of carcinogen metabolism genes and risk of squamous cell carcinoma of the head and neck. Head Neck 2007;29:682–99.

[7] D'Souza G, Kreimer AR, Viscidi R, et al. Case-control study of human papillomavirus and oropharyngeal cancer. N Engl J Med 2007;356:1944–56.

[8] Kreimer AR, Clifford GM, Boyle P, et al. Human papillomavirus types in head and neck squamous cell carcinomas worldwide: a systematic review. Cancer Epidemiol Biomarkers Prev 2005;14:467–75.

[9] Ragin CC, Modugno F, Gollin SM. The epidemiology and risk factors of head and neck cancer: a focus on human papillomavirus. J Dent Res 2007;86:104–14.

[10] Manjarrez ME, Ocadiz R, Valle L, et al. Detection of human papillomavirus and relevant tumor suppressors and oncoproteins in laryngeal tumors. Clin Cancer Res 2006;12: 6946–51.

[11] Hobbs CG, Sterne JA, Bailey M, et al. Human papillomavirus and head and neck cancer: a systematic review and meta-analysis. Clin Otolaryngol 2006;31:259–66.

[12] Wiatrak BJ, Wiatrak DW, Broker TR, et al. Recurrent respiratory papillomatosis: a longitudinal study comparing severity associated with human papilloma viral types 6 and 11 and other risk factors in a large pediatric population. Laryngoscope 2004;114:1–23.

[13] Lele SM, Pou AM, Ventura K, et al. Molecular events in the progression of recurrent respiratory papillomatosis to carcinoma. Arch Pathol Lab Med 2002;126:1184–8.

[14] Rady PL, Schnadig VJ, Weiss R, et al. Malignant transformation of recurrent respiratory papillomatosis associated with integrated human papillomavirus type 11 DNA and mutation of p53. Laryngoscope 1998;108:735–40.

[15] Knudson AG Jr. Mutation and cancer: statistical study of retinoblastoma. Proc Natl Acad Sci USA 1971;68:820–3.

[16] Fearon ER, Vogelstein B. A genetic model for colorectal tumorigenesis. Cell 1990;1:759–67.

[17] Califano J, van der Riet P, Westra W, et al. Genetic progression model for head and neck cancer: implications for field cancerization. Cancer Res 1996;56:2488–92.

[18] Gollin SM. Chromosomal alterations in squamous cell carcinomas of the head and neck: window to the biology of disease. Head Neck 2001;23:238–53.

[19] Carey TE, Van Dyke DL, Worsham MJ. Nonrandom chromosome aberrations and clonal populations in head and neck cancer. Anticancer Res 1993;13:2561–7.

[20] Jin Y, Mertens F, Mandahl N, et al. Chromosome abnormalities in eighty-three head and neck squamous cell carcinomas: influence of culture conditions on karyotypic pattern. Cancer Res 1993;53:2140–6.

[21] Jin Y, Mertens F. Chromosome abnormalities in oral squamous cell carcinomas. Eur J Cancer B Oral Oncol 1993;29:257–63.

[22] Rosin MP, Cheng X, Poh C, et al. Use of allelic loss to predict malignant risk for low-grade oral epithelial dysplasia. Clin Cancer Res 2000;6:357–62.

[23] Bosch FX, Ritter D, Enders C, et al. Head and neck tumor sites differ in prevalence and spectrum of p53 alterations but these have limited prognostic value. Int J Cancer 2004; 111:530–8.

[24] Wang Q, Han D, Wang W. Adenovirus-mediated p53 gene therapy of human laryngeal cancer. Zhonghua Zhong Liu Za Zhi 1998;20:418–21.

[25] Qiu Z, Lao M, Wu C. Co-transfer of human wild-type p53 and granulocyte-macrophage colony-stimulating factor genes via recombinant adenovirus induces apoptosis and enhances immunogenicity in laryngeal cancer cells. Cancer Lett 2001;167:25–32.

[26] Qiu ZH, Wu CT, Lao MF, et al. Growth suppression and immunogenicity enhancement of hep-2 or primary laryngeal cancer cells by adenovirus-mediated co-transfer of human wild-type p53, granulocyte-macrophage colony-stimulating factor and B7-1 genes. Cancer Lett 2002;182:147–54.

[27] Reed AL, Califano J, Cairns P, et al. High frequency of p16 (CDKN2/MTS-1/INK4A) inactivation in head and neck squamous cell carcinoma. Cancer Res 1996;56:3630–3.

[28] Akanuma D, Uzawa N, Yoshida MA, et al. Inactivation patterns of the p16(INK4a) gene in oral squamous cell carcinoma cell lines. Oral Oncol 1999;35:476–83.

[29] Hasegawa M, Nelson HH, Peters E, et al. Patterns of gene promoter methylation in squamous cell cancer of the head and neck. Oncogene 2002;21:4231–6.

[30] Riese U, Dahse R, Fiedler W, et al. Tumor suppressor gene p16 (CDKN2A) mutation status and promoter inactivation in head and neck cancer. Int J Mol Med 1999;4:61–5.

[31] Ha P, Califano JA. Promoter methylation and inactivation of tumour-suppressor genes in oral squamous-cell carcinoma. Lancet Oncol 2006;7:77–82.

[32] Calmon MF, Colombo J, Carvalho F, et al. Methylation profile of genes CDKN2A (p14 and p16), DAPK1, CDH1, and ADAM23 in head and neck cancer. Cancer Genet Cytogenet 2007;173:31–7.

[33] Temam S, Bénard J, Dugas C, et al. Molecular detection of early-stage laryngopharyngeal squamous cell carcinomas. Clin Cancer Res 2005;11:2547–51.

[34] Smith IM, Mydlarz WK, Mithani SK, et al. DNA global hypomethylation in squamous cell head and neck cancer associated with smoking, alcohol consumption and stage. Int J Cancer 2007;121:1724–8.

[35] Dassonville O, Formento JL, Francoual M, et al. Expression of epidermal growth factor receptor and survival in upper aerodigestive tract cancer. J Clin Oncol 1993;11: 1873–8.

[36] Kalyankrishna S, Grandis JR. Epidermal growth factor receptor biology in head and neck cancer. J Clin Oncol 2006;24:2666–72.

[37] Santini J, Formento JL, Francoual M, et al. Characterization, quantification, and potential clinical value of the epidermal growth factor receptor in head and neck squamous cell carcinomas. Head Neck 1991;13:132–9.

[38] Lothaire P, Azambuja Ed, Dequanter D, et al. Molecular markers of head and neck squamous cell carcinoma: promising signs in need of prospective evaluation. Head Neck 2006;28:256–69.

[39] O-Charoenrat P, Rhys-Evans PH, Modjtahedi H, et al. The role of c-erbB receptors and ligands in head and neck squamous cell carcinoma. Oral Oncol 2002;38:627–40.

[40] Imai K, Takaoka A. Comparing antibody and small-molecule therapies for cancer. Nat Rev Cancer 2006;6:714–27.

[41] Loeffler-Ragg J, Witsch-Baumgartner M, Tzankov A, et al. Low incidence of mutations in EGFR kinase domain in Caucasian patients with head and neck squamous cell carcinoma. Eur J Cancer 2006;42:109–11.

[42] Demiral AN, Sarioglu S, Birlik B, et al. Prognostic significance of EGF receptor expression in early glottic cancer. Auris Nasus Larynx 2004;31:417–24.

[43] Kawaguchi Y, Kono K, Mimura K, et al. Cetuximab induces antibody-dependent cellular cytotoxicity against EGFR-expressing esophageal squamous cell carcinoma. Int J Cancer 2007;120:781–7.

[44] Trigo R, Hitt P, Koralewski E, et al. Cetuximab monotherapy is active in patients (pts) with platinum-refractory recurrent/metastatic squamous cell carcinoma of the head and neck (SCCHN): results of a phase II study. J Clin Oncol 2004;22:5502 [Meeting abstracts].

[45] Robert F, Ezekiel MP, Spencer SA, et al. Phase I study of anti-epidermal growth factor receptor antibody cetuximab in combination with radiation therapy in patients with advanced head and neck cancer. J Clin Oncol 2001;19:3234–43.

[46] Burtness B, Goldwasser MA, Flood W, et al. Phase III randomized trial of cisplatin plus placebo compared with cisplatin plus cetuximab in metastatic/recurrent head and neck cancer: an Eastern Cooperative Oncology Group study. J Clin Oncol 2005;23:8646–54.

[47] Bonner JA, Harari PM, Giralt J, et al. Improved preservation of larynx with the addition of cetuximab to radiation for cancers of the larynx and hypopharynx. J Clin Oncol 2005;23: 5533 [Meeting abstracts].

[48] Bonner JA, Harari PM, Giralt J, et al. Radiotherapy plus cetuximab for squamous-cell carcinoma of the head and neck. N Engl J Med 2006;354:567–78.

[49] Robert F, Blumenschein G, Herbst RS, et al. Phase I/IIa study of cetuximab with gemcitabine plus carboplatin in patients with chemotherapy-naive advanced non-small-cell lung cancer. J Clin Oncol 2005;23:9089–96.

[50] Shin DM, Donato NJ, Perez-Soler R, et al. Epidermal growth factor receptor-targeted therapy with C225 and cisplatin in patients with head and neck cancer. Clin Cancer Res 2001;7:1204–13.

[51] American Society of Clinical Oncology, Pfister DG, Laurie SA, et al. American Society of Clinical Oncology clinical practice guideline for the use of larynx—preservation strategies in the treatment of laryngeal cancer. J Clin Oncol 2006;24:3693–704.

[52] De La Garza G, Granados M, Aguilar JL, et al. Phase II clinical trial preliminary report: cetuximab, gemcitabine and simultaneous radiotherapy for locally advanced head and neck cancer: preliminary report. J Clin Oncol 2006 ASCO Annual Meeting Proceedings (Post-Meeting Edition) 2006;24:15502.

[53] Cohen EE. Role of epidermal growth factor receptor pathway-targeted therapy in patients with recurrent and/or metastatic squamous cell carcinoma of the head and neck. J Clin Oncol 2006;24:2659–65.

[54] Siu LL, Soulieres D, Chen EX, et al. Phase I/II trial of erlotinib and cisplatin in patients with recurrent or metastatic squamous cell carcinoma of the head and neck: a Princess Margaret Hospital phase II consortium and National Cancer Institute of Canada Clinical Trials Group Study. J Clin Oncol 2007;25:2178–83.

[55] Matar P, Rojo F, Cassia R, et al. Combined epidermal growth factor receptor targeting with the tyrosine kinase inhibitor gefitinib (ZD1839) and the monoclonal antibody cetuximab (IMC-C225): superiority over single-agent receptor targeting. Clin Cancer Res 2004;10: 6487–501.

[56] Baselga J, Schoffski P, Rojo H, et al. A phase I pharmacokinetic (PK) and molecular pharmacodynamic (PD) study of the combination of two anti-EGFR therapies, the monoclonal antibody (MAb) cetuximab (C) and the tyrosine kinase inhibitor (TKI) gefitinib (G), in patients (pts) with advanced colorectal (CRC), head and neck (HNC) and non-small cell lung cancer (NSCLC). ASCO Annual Meeting Proceedings 2006;24:3006.

[57] Prenzel N, Zwick E, Daub H, et al. EGF receptor transactivation by G-protein-coupled receptors requires metalloproteinase cleavage of proHB-EGF. Nature 1999;402:884–8.

[58] Cohen EE, Lingen MW, Martin LE, et al. Response of some head and neck cancers to epidermal growth factor receptor tyrosine kinase inhibitors may be linked to mutation of ERBB2 rather than EGFR. Clin Cancer Res 2005;11:8105–8.

[59] Nelson AR, Rothenberg ML. Matrix metalloproteinases: biologic activity and clinical implications. J Clin Oncol 2000;18:1135–49.

[60] Kerrebijn JDF, Simons PJ, Tas M, et al. The effects of thymostimulin on immunological function in patients with head and neck cancer. Clin Otolaryngol 1996;21:455–62.

[61] Coussens LM, Werb Z. Matrix metalloproteinases and the development of cancer. Chem Biol 1996;3:895–904.

[62] Garraud O, Faucher A, Legrand E, et al. Impairment of monocyte functions in advanced head and neck cancer. Immunol Lett 1988;18:213–8.

[63] Muraki Y, Yoshioka C, Tateishi A, et al. Localization of Fas antigen in oral squamous cell carcinoma. Br J Oral Maxillofac Surg 1999;37:37–40.

[64] Peschos D, Damala C, Stefanou D, et al. Expression of matrix metalloproteinase-9 (gelatinase B) in benign, premalignant and malignant laryngeal lesions. Histol Histopathol 2006;21:603–8.

[65] Lee JW, Soung YH, Kim SY, et al. Somatic mutations of EGFR gene in squamous cell carcinoma of the head and neck. Clin Cancer Res 2005;11:2879–82.

[66] Liu WW, Zeng ZY, Wu QL, et al. Overexpression of MMP-2 in laryngeal squamous cell carcinoma: a potential indicator for poor prognosis. Otolaryngol Head Neck Surg 2005; 132:395–400.

[67] Smith BD, Smith BL, Carter D, et al. Prognostic significance of vascular endothelial growth factor protein levels in oral and oropharyngeal squamous cell carcinoma. J Clin Oncol 2000; 18:2046–52.

[68] Kyzas PA, Cunha IW, Ioannidis PA, et al. Prognostic significance of vascular endothelial growth factor immunohistochemical expression in head and neck squamous cell carcinoma: a meta-analysis. Clin Cancer Res 2005;11:1434–40.

[69] Hinojar-Gutierrez A, Fernandez-Contreras ME, Gonzalez-Gonzalez R, et al. Intratumoral lymphatic vessels and VEGF-C expression are predictive factors of lymph node relapse in T1-T4 NO laryngopharyngeal squamous cell carcinoma. Ann Surg Oncol 2007;14:248–57.

[70] Letessier EM, Sacchi M, Johnson JT, et al. The absence of lymphoid suppressor cells in tumor-involved lymph nodes of patients with head and neck cancer. Cell Immunol 1990; 130:446–58.

[71] Kong HL, Hecht D, Song W, et al. Regional suppression of tumor growth by in vivo transfer of a cDNA encoding a secreted form of the extracellular domain of the flt-1 vascular endothelial growth factor receptor. Hum Gene Ther 1998;9:823–933.

[72] Whiteside TL, Chikamatsu K, Nagashima S. Antitumor effects of cytolytic T lymphocytes (CTL) and natural killer (NK) cells in head and neck cancer. Anticancer Res 1996;16: 2357–64.

[73] Vlock DR. Immunobiologic aspects of head and neck cancer. Clinical and laboratory correlates. Hematol Oncol Clin North Am 1991;5:797–820.

[74] Hald J, Rasmussen N, Claesson MH. Tumour-infiltrating lymphocytes mediate lysis of autologous squamous cell carcinomas of the head and neck. Cancer Immunol Immunother 1995;41:243–50.

[75] Pries R, Wollenberg B. Cytokines in head and neck cancer. Cytokine Growth Factor Rev 2006;17:141–6.

[76] Tas MP, Simons PJ, Balm FJ, et al. Depressed monocyte polarization and clustering of dendritic cells in patients with head and neck cancer: in vitro restoration of this immunosuppression by thymic hormones. Cancer Immunol Immunother 1993;36:108–14.

[77] Westermarck J, Kahari VM. Regulation of matrix metalloproteinase expression in tumor invasion. FASEB J 1999;13:781–92.

[78] Cameron DJ, Stromberg BV. The ability of macrophages from head and neck cancer patients to kill tumor cells. Effect of prostaglandin inhibitors on cytotoxicity. Cancer 1984;54:2403–8.

[79] McCawley LJ, Crawford HC, King LE, et al. A protective role for matrix metalloproteinase-3 in squamous cell carcinoma. Cancer Res 2004;64:6965–72.

[80] Kerrebijn JD, Balm AJ, Freeman JL, et al. Who is in control of the immune system in head and neck cancer? Crit Rev Oncol Hematol 1999;31:31–53.

[81] Sundelin K, Jadner M, Norberg-Spaak L, et al. Metallothionein and Fas (CD95) are expressed in squamous cell carcinoma of the tongue. Eur J Cancer 1997;33:1860–4.

[82] Kim JW, Wieckowski E, Taylor DD, et al. Fas ligand-positive membranous vesicles isolated from sera of patients with oral cancer induce apoptosis of activated T lymphocytes. Clin Cancer Res 2005;11:1010–20.

[83] Airoldi M, De Stefani A, Marchionatti S, et al. Survival in patients with recurrent squamous cell head and neck carcinoma treated with bio-chemotherapy. Head Neck 2001;23:298–304.

[84] Cortesina G, De Stefani A, Galeazzi E, et al. Interleukin-2 injected around tumor-draining lymph nodes in head and neck cancer. Head Neck 1991;13:125–31.

[85] Bray D, Yu SZ, Koprowski H II, et al. Combination nonviral interleukin 2 gene therapy and external-beam radiation therapy for head and neck cancer. Arch Otolaryngol Head Neck Surg 2003;129:618–22.

[86] Xian J, Yang H, Lin Y, et al. Combination nonviral murine interleukin 2 and interleukin 12 gene therapy and radiotherapy for head and neck squamous cell carcinoma. Arch Otolaryngol Head Neck Surg 2005;131:1079–85.

[87] Kimura Y, Tojima H, Fukase S, et al. Clinical evaluation of sizofilan as assistant immunotherapy in treatment of head and neck cancer. Acta Otolaryngol Suppl 1994;511:192–5.

[88] Fukazawa H, Ohashi Y, Sekiyama S, et al. Multidisciplinary treatment of head and neck cancer using BCG, OK-432, and GE-132 as biologic response modifiers. Head Neck 1994; 16:30–8.

[89] Monji M, Senju S, Nakatsura T, et al. Head and neck cancer antigens recognized by the humoral immune system. Biochem Biophys Res Commun 2002;294:734–41.

ELSEVIER
SAUNDERS

Otolaryngol Clin N Am
41 (2008) 673–695

OTOLARYNGOLOGIC
CLINICS
OF NORTH AMERICA

Laryngeal Cancer: Diagnosis and Preoperative Work-up

Eugene A. Chu, MD, Young J. Kim, MD, PhD*

Department of Otolaryngology, Head and Neck Surgery, Johns Hopkins University School of Medicine, 6210 JHOC, 601 North Caroline Street, Baltimore, MD 21287-0910, USA

Laryngeal carcinoma is the eleventh-most common form of cancer among men worldwide and is the second-most common malignancy of the head and neck. In the United States in 2007 there were an estimated 11,300 new cases of laryngeal cancer and 3,600 cases of disease-specific mortality [1]. The primary functions of the larynx involve phonation, respiration, and deglutition but it also contributes to taste and smell by allowing the movement of air over the special sense organs. Thus, loss of laryngeal function affects speech and swallowing and some of the senses that allow us to enjoy the world. Moreover, total laryngectomy bypasses the critical humidification function of the upper aerodigestive tract that renders pulmonary toiletry problematic for these patients. With relatively little change in mortality since the 1970s, recent research has focused not only on improving survival but on laryngeal preservation modalities.

Prevention and early diagnosis of laryngeal carcinoma is the most effective means for maximizing cure rates and preserving function. Fortunately, glottic laryngeal carcinoma, the most common laryngeal tumor, tends to be detected at an earlier stage than tumors located at other subsites of the head and neck. Nevertheless, the symptoms of laryngeal carcinoma can also be nonspecific and may result in a delay of diagnosis. In general, hoarseness lasting longer than 3 weeks or odynophagia or dysphagia lasting longer than 6 weeks should warrant a referral to an otolaryngologist—especially for patients older than 50 years with an extensive smoking or drinking history. Associated otalgia, stridor, and weight loss should also be red flags to completely rule out a malignant process.

The preoperative evaluation of patients with laryngeal carcinoma begins with a thorough history and physical examination in the office with

---

* Corresponding author.

E-mail address: ykim76@gw.johnshopkins.edu (Y.J. Kim).

0030-6665/08/$ - see front matter © 2008 Elsevier Inc. All rights reserved.
doi:10.1016/j.otc.2008.01.016

subsequent endoscopy and surgical biopsy for tissue diagnosis. Once a diagnosis is made, the physician and patient must together formulate an individualized plan based on the tumor characteristics as well as the patient's wishes. In McNeil's frequently quoted study of firemen and upper management executives with advanced laryngeal cancer, one of five patients would accept a 20% to 30% decrease in survival to preserve their voice [2]. This study clearly demonstrates that patients place a significant premium on quality of life and that clinicians cannot perseverate on maximizing survival alone. Another critical issue in the formulation of a treatment plan is an open discussion regarding some of the recent findings of short-term and long-term quality of life in patients who have undergone partial and total laryngectomies as well as endoscopic partial laryngectomies.

Biology of laryngeal malignancy

Effective treatment and understanding of laryngeal cancer requires fundamental knowledge of the complex anatomy of this region. Based on its embryologic development, the larynx can be divided into three levels: supraglottic, glottic, and subglottic, with each level containing a number of subsites (Table 1). These divisions have clinical relevance in that they help predict the clinical behavior and pattern of spread of the tumor.

The supraglottis extends from the tip of the epiglottis superiorly to the apices of the ventricles and undersurface of the false cords and includes both the lingual and laryngeal surfaces of the epiglottis, the arytenoid cartilages, the aryepiglottic (AE) folds, and the false cords. The supraglottis develops from the midline buccopharyngeal anlage from branchial arches 4 and 6 with rich bilateral lymphatics. Clinically, this translates to a significant incidence of unilateral or bilateral cervical metastasis—25% to 75% for all T-stages [3,4].

The glottic larynx encompasses the floor of the ventricle, the true vocal folds extending to 0.5 cm below the free edge of the cord, the anterior commisure, and the interarytenoid area. In contrast to the supraglottic structures, the glottis forms from the midline fusion of lateral structures derived from the

Table 1
Anatomic levels and subsites of the larynx

Level	Subsites
Supraglottis	Suprahyoid epiglottis (tip, lingual, and laryngeal surfaces)
	Aryepiglottic fold
	Arytenoids
	Infrahyoid epiglottis
	False cords
Glottis	True vocal folds
	Anterior commisure
	Posterior commisure
Subglottis	

tracheobronchial anlage from arches 4, 5, and 6 and has a relative dearth of lymphatics. Consequently, this embryologic boundary limits submucosal spread to adjacent sites within the larynx for early stage cancers, and the paucity of lymphatic in the glottis contains lymphatic spread to the neck allowing glottic cancers to remain localized to the larynx for longer periods of time.

The subglottis continues from the inferior limit of the glottis to the inferior edge of the cricoid cartilage. It develops from the fourth and sixth pharyngeal arches and because of its location has a propensity for extralaryngeal extension.

Laryngeal framework

Except for advance stage tumors, most laryngeal cancers tend to remain confined to one anatomic site because of the "pushing" mechanism of tumor growth (Fig. 1). Seminal dye and histologic studies have confirmed this compartmentalization in lymphatics and vasculature [5,6]. Additionally, cartilaginous and fascial anatomic structures, such as the thyroid and cricoid cartilages with their overlying perichondrium, the ventricle, the conus elasticus, the quadrangular and thyrohyoid membranes, and the hyoepiglottic ligament, act as barriers to spread (Fig. 2). The anterior commisure and thyrohyoid membrane, in contradistinction to the above structures, offers little resistance to tumor spread. For the purpose of TNM staging, knowledge of these anatomic ligaments and potential spaces may not be helpful; however, in the overall evaluation of laryngeal malignancy, framing the work-up of the lesion in the context of these barriers is critical in providing the optimal diagnosis and therapy for the patient.

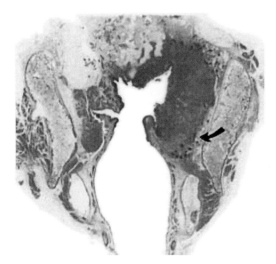

Fig. 1. Broad "pushing" margins of a supraglottic tumor that does not violate the glottis. (*From* Thawley et al. Comprehensive Management of Head & Neck Tumors. 2nd ed.)

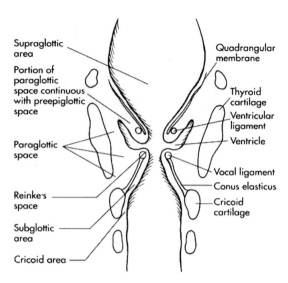

Fig. 2. Fascial planes of the larynx and the potential spaces created by these anatomic barriers. (*From* Cummings, et al. Otolaryngology: Head & Neck Surgery. 4th ed.)

Laryngeal spaces (potential)

Pre-epiglottic space

These fibroelastic membranes and ligaments define two critical potential spaces around the larynx. The pre-epiglottic space is bound superiorly by the hyoepiglottic ligament, anteriorly by the thyroid cartilage and thyrohyoid membrane, and posteriorly by the epiglottis and thyroepiglottic ligament. The cartilage of the epiglottis has numerous perforations that allow transit of tumor from the posterior surface of the epiglottis into the pre-epiglottic space. Furthermore, dehiscences in the thyrohyoid membrane created by the superior laryngeal neurovascular bundle allow extension of tumor from the pre-epiglottic space into the neck.

Paraglottic space

Alternatively, tumor may invade in a cephalad-caudal spread via the paraglottic space into all the subsites of the larynx (Fig. 3). The paraglottis space is a potential space, and together with the pre-epiglottic space forms, a horseshoe-shaped fatty space around the internal laryngeal structures. The lateral boundaries of the paraglottic space are the thyroid cartilage anteriorly and the mucosa overlying the medial wall of the piriform sinus posteriorly. Superiorly and medially lie the quadrangular membrane, and the conus elasticus is situated inferiorly. Involvement of the paraglottic space by tumor allows fascial free access to the supraglottic, glottic, and subglottic regions in addition to the soft tissues of the neck. Transglottic tumors by definition involve the paraglottic space superior and inferior to the ventricle (see Fig. 3).

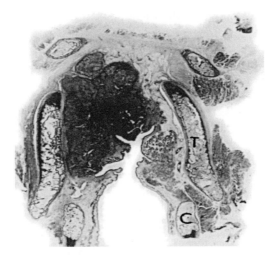

Fig. 3. Supraglottic tumor through the paraglottic space rendering the tumor transglottic. (*From* Cummings, et al. Otolaryngology: Head & Neck Surgery. 4th ed.)

Office evaluation

The are three major goals to the initial evaluation:

(1) Determining whether or not the lesion is malignant (tissue diagnosis)
(2) Staging the lesion in the context of the optimal treatment for the patient
(3) Mapping both the gross disease and regional nodes as well as potential occult or metastatic disease.

The typical patient is a male in his 50s or 60s with a history of smoking and alcohol use. However, the male predilection for this disease has recently decreased from a male:female ratio of 15:1 to currently less than 5:1 [7]. This change in demographics has been attributed to increased rates of smoking among females and their increasing presence in equally toxic work environments. Significant variation in the distribution of carcinoma at the different laryngeal subsites exists worldwide. Supraglottic and glottic tumors are the most prominent subsites, and subglottic carcinomas are uniformly rare. In the United States, glottic carcinomas are the most common (glottic, 59%; supraglottic, 40%; subglottic, 1%) [7,8]. However, given the heterogeneity of ethnic and immigrant population in the North American cities, clinical suspicion for uncommon subsites as well as risk factors related to ethnic diet and customs should be considered.

History

As with all head and neck malignancies, the evaluation begins with a thorough history. This should include not only a careful review of the chief complaint but also an assessment of associated medical problems, social history (specifically amount and duration of tobacco and alcohol use), family history of all types of malignancies, and a complete review of symptoms with an eye toward any symptoms suggestive of metastatic involvement. Careful review of the patient's history and symptoms can often give insight into the location and extent of the disease.

Typical symptoms include hoarseness, dysphagia, odynophagia, neck mass, referred otalgia, dyspnea, and aspiration. Since minor changes to the vocal fold affect the mucosal wave and result in hoarseness, it comes as no surprise that glottic tumors tend to be diagnosed at an earlier stage than supraglottic or subglottic cancers. Hoarseness in the latter two instances would suggest a more advanced lesion with spread to either the cricoarytenoid unit or deep invasion into the laryngeal musculature. It is important to note that patients with reflux laryngitis and heavy smoking history may have a chronically inflamed larynx at baseline and may not appreciate subtle changes in their voice. Dyspnea could be a result of either significant vocal fold motion impairment or bulky disease while dysphagia and odynophagia suggest possible involvement of the tongue base or hypopharynx.

Supraglottic tumors

In contrast to glottic tumors, supraglottic tumors often come to the attention of a head and neck surgeon only after persistent symptoms of dysphagia, odynophagia, and otalgia. Because of the nonspecific nature of their symptoms, these patients have frequently already seen other physicians who have treated them with medical therapies without a clear diagnosis. At the time of presentation, many patients have already developed palpable neck disease and significant weight loss.

Subglottic tumors are rare and often present in the emergent setting with airway obstruction or vocal fold paralysis. Hypopharyngeal malignancies, which are less common in the United States, also present as advanced disease with comparable symptoms as supraglottic lesions with related risk factors such as tobacco use and extensive alcohol use. Aside from postcricoid carcinoma, hypopharyngeal tumors also present in men with a heavy smoking and drinking history. Women of European descent with chronic dysphagia and history of Plummer-Vinson syndrome should also be a red flag in the evaluation for hypopharyngeal lesions, particularly postcricoid subsite.

Etiology

Tobacco and alcohol abuse

Eighty-five percent of laryngeal cancers can be attributed to tobacco and alcohol use. Smoking is the predominant risk factor for laryngeal carcinoma with alcohol use being an independent and synergistic risk factor [9].

Current smokers have a 10- to 20-fold increased risk of laryngeal cancer compared with nonsmokers [10,11]. However, these risks decline sharply after smoking cessation—although never to the same level as patients who have never smoked. Ten to 15 years after smoking cessation, there is an approximately 60% reduction in relative risk. While smoking cessation is the single most effective means of preventing laryngeal cancer, it is equally important to encourage patients to quit smoking after the diagnosis of laryngeal cancer has been made. Smoking has been identified as an independent risk factor for local recurrence and for recurrence at an earlier time point than those who ceased smoking [12].

Other risk factors include carcinogens in the workplace such as asbestos, nickel compounds, wood dust, leather products, paint, diesel fume, and glass-wool [13]. Additionally, there is a controversial association with chronic gastroesophageal reflux [14] as well as an increased incidence of squamous cell carcinoma in preexisting laryngeal respiratory papillomatosis. While there is good evidence for a causal link between human papillomavirus (HPV) subtypes 16 and 18 and oropharyngeal cancer, the association with laryngeal cancer is not as robust [15,16].

Comprehensive medical history

Patients with a prior history of a head and neck malignancy have an approximately 14% chance of developing a second primary malignancy in the head and neck. It is important to review the patient's past medical history not only for prior malignancies but also for conditions that may warrant extra preoperative work-up, ie, significant coronary artery disease or chronic obstructive pulmonary lung disease. Clinical pulmonary function assessment is critical in the choice of treatment since baseline pulmonary reserve partly dictates the success of conservation laryngeal surgery. An assessment of the patient's motor ability helps predict the likelihood of success with a tracheo-esophageal prosthesis for voicing. Additionally, based on the patient's history and examination, nutrition and dental consultation should be considered as needed.

Finally, the patient's social history should be considered in as much as it can influence treatment decisions. For example, two patients with identical-stage tumors but one whose livelihood is dependent on his or her voice and the other a patient who is a social recluse with limited transportation capability, may each benefit from different treatment plans. According to the preeminent clinician, Osler, this is a classic situation where the physician should "treat the patient," and not the disease.

Physical examination

The overall goals of the office examination are to assess the extent of tumor involvement, vocal cord mobility, airway patency, and the extent of locoregional spread. To this end, a complete head and neck examination, including examination of all mucosal surfaces, is essential, especially given the 4% to 8% incidence of synchronous lesions in upper aero-digestive tract in patients with head and neck malignancies. Visualization of the larynx by either mirror and/or endoscopic examination is mandatory.

All regions above the clavicle are carefully palpated for evidence of metastatic disease or direct extralaryngeal extension. All too often, clinical examination on the lateral aspect of the neck is extensively documented without a careful assessment of the midline structures. Loss of the normal crepitance with side-to-side movement of the laryngeal framework may indicate postcricoid involvement. Complete fixation of the laryngeal complex on clinical examination is also suggestive of prevertebral involvement. Careful palpable assessment of the thyrohyoid membrane, thyroid cartilage, and cricothryoid membrane, as well as the overlying soft tissue of the laryngeal complex may provide a more clinically useful assessment of the tumor than any advanced imaging analysis. Laryngeal carcinoma most frequently metastasizes to nodal levels II, III, and IV in the neck. Supraglottic tumors have the highest rates of occult cervical metastasis: T1, 20%; T2, 40%; T3, 60%; and T4, 80%. Early glottic lesions have a less than 7% incidence of occult metastasis but T4 lesions can have up to a 40% incidence [17,18]. Physical examination directed toward central compartment lymphatic spread (Delphian nodes) must not be ignored. Subglottic tumors have a significant incidence of extralaryngeal spread because of their proximity to the cricothyroid membrane and the rich postcricoid lymphatics. However, the true incidence of occult metastasis for subglottic disease is difficult to determine because of the rarity of the disease.

Pulmonary status

The patient's pulmonary status will help determine the timing of planned surgical endoscopy and the need for possible tumor debulking versus tracheostomy. Audible stridor and use of accessory muscles during breathing at rest may require an urgent or emergent surgical airway. Pulmonary function tests and a careful review of the patient's exercise tolerance (ie, can he or she walk up two flight of stairs without stopping?) are especially important if conservation surgery is being contemplated because the patient's preoperative pulmonary reserve is an important indicator of how well the patient will tolerate aspiration postoperatively. Nevertheless, no objective standards exist that can reliably distinguish which patients are able to tolerate the physiologic changes accompanying conservation laryngeal surgery.

Laryngoscopy

Office-based laryngoscopy should answer several questions. First and foremost is to look for any lesions. The critical sites to evaluate are base of tongue, valleculae, epiglottis, aryepiglottic folds, arytenoids, interarytenoid regions, false cords, ventricles (if possible), true cords, subglottis (if possible), and some of the subsites of the hypopharynx. Extensive pooling of saliva in the piriform sinus and the larynx should be noted as a subtle sign for other occult pathology. Last, laryngoscopy should be used to assess the gross appearance and growth pattern (exophytic versus submucosal) since this may raise the suspicion for skip lesions, occult disease, subclinically extensive tumor, or nonsquamous pathology.

Indirect mirror laryngoscopy provides an excellent overview of the larynx and tongue base as well as excellent color and depth perception. However, it is often difficult to visualize the anterior commisure, especially in patients with a strong gag reflex.

Flexible fiber-optic laryngoscopy (FFL), possibly combined with strobo-scopy, allows a closer look at individual areas and allows for video and pho-tographic documentation of any visible pathology in a physiologic setting. Patients often appreciate being able to directly visualize the lesion on the monitor and it may facilitate their understanding of the disease process. The office examination provides the best opportunity to assess vocal fold movement as well as movement of the cricoarytenoid joint. Maneuvers, such as having the patient cough lightly, may help elucidate arytenoid mobility or lack thereof.

It is critical to distinguish between a true fixed vocal fold due to paraglot-tic space invasion versus cricoarytenoid joint involvement by the tumor. Bilateral arytenoid immobility secondary to cricoarytenoid involvement with tumor is a contraindication to organ preservation surgery. The extent of the tumor or suspicious areas for biopsy will aid the planning of the operative laryngoscopy and biopsy. With adequate topical anesthesia, the flexible fiber-optic laryngoscope can be passed through the cords to visualize the subglottis. Evaluation of the patency of the airway combined with vocal fold function can prevent unforeseen difficulties with subsequent intubation.

Rigid endoscopic evaluation

Rigid 70° or 90° endoscopes provide a similar view as with indirect mirror laryngoscopy but with added magnification. Similar to FFL, rigid endo-scopes when combined with a stroboscopic light source allows for excellent visualization of the mucosal wave and may aid in detecting early glottic lesions by subtle changes in mucosal wave dynamics. Extrusion of the tongue required for rigid endoscopy may place the larynx in a slight non-physiologic position, but the wealth of clinical information it provides outweighs theoretic arguments against its use. The practical worries of patients with strong gag reflex can be resolved with practical experience.

The current standard of care calls for biopsies in the operating room dur-ing surgical endoscopy; however, sheaths with working channels are now available that fit over existing flexible fiber-optic laryngoscopes allowing for in-office transnasal endoscopic biopsies (MedtronicENT, Inc, Jackson-ville, Florida). In fact, use of transnasal laryngoscopy and esophagoscopy may facilitate or substitute the operative panendoscopy in select cancer patients. In a prospective study of 17 patients, Postma and colleagues [19] found transnasal endoscopic biopsy results to be entirely congruent with standard panendoscopy biopsies taken in the operating room. The biopsies obtained via transnasal endoscopy were diagnostic for cancer in 12 of 12 patients and negative for malignancy in 5 of 5.

TNM staging dictates that true vocal cord mobility is properly assessed for proper staging according to American Joint Committee on Cancer (AJCC). However, it should be highlighted that the cricoarytenoid unit is the basic functional unit of the hemilarynx, and the visible abnormal mobility of the true cords should be assessed with this in mind. The function of the cricoarytenoid unit dictates whether the patient is a candidate for organ preservation surgery. The fixation of the involved cords on office-based laryngoscopy may stage the patients as T3, but this does not sufficiently assist in the treatment plan. Furthermore, the possibility of pseudofixation because of bulky mass effect on the arytenoids should be assessed whenever possible.

Imaging

Imaging serves as a critical adjunct to the physical examination, and not a substitute. It can be useful for staging. Imaging can provide valuable assessment of anatomic spaces difficult to objectively assess on physical examination or by endoscopy (pre-epiglottic space, paraglottic space, thyroid cartilage invasion). Imaging may also supplement clinical examination information as to the tumor volume and extralaryngeal extension. Furthermore, imaging can assist with surgical planning and in the determination of whether or not the primary tumor is amenable to resection [20]. A more detailed account of imaging in laryngeal malignancy is available in the article by Blitz and Aygun, elsewhere in this issue.

CT versus MRI

Computed tomography (CT) or magnetic resonance imaging (MRI) of the head and neck from the skull base to clavicles are both appropriate initial imaging choices. T2-weighted MRI allows for excellent visualization of subtle submucosal spread into the pre-epiglottic and paraglottic spaces. Extensive pre-epiglottic fat invasion places the hyoid bone at risk for involvement, which has implications for some laryngeal conservation procedures that sometimes require the hyoid as part of the closure. Paraglottic space involvement increases the risk of neck disease and cartilage invasion. The degree, if any, of laryngeal cartilage invasion is also critical to surgical planning. While minor cartilaginous invasion (staged as T3) is now being treated with chemoradiation protocols, through-and-through cartilage invasion is an indication for surgical resection of the larynx because of the high incidence of chondronecrosis after radiation.

CT has a higher specificity but lower sensitivity for thyroid cartilage invasion when compared with MRI [21–23]. Nevertheless, both have comparable accuracy rates—75% to 80% and 80% to 85%, respectively [20]. Palpation for cervical lymph node metastasis has a 25% to 51% false-negative rate [17], while substantial literature demonstrates an 87% to 93% accuracy in CT staging of the neck [24]. Although fewer reports support its use, MRI has been reported as having comparable results to CT in evaluation of the neck [24]. Imaging can also aid in determining whether or not a lesion is amenable to resection by assessing for vascular encasement, prevertebral fascia involvement, or mediastinal involvement—factors that would make a lesion T4b and therefore considered unresectable [20,25,26].

Role of PET/CT

The role of fused modality positron emission tomography/computed tomography (PET/CT) in diagnosing and staging patients with primary metastasis and recurrent head and neck cancer has been evolving. PET/CT combines the detailed anatomic information of the CT with PET's ability to detect subtle lesions by alterations in metabolic activity. Several studies have confirmed its utility in the pretreatment period. Fleming and colleagues [27] in a study of 123 patients with known head and neck cancer found that use of pretreatment PET/CT imaging changed management in 30.9% of the patients. These results are in agreement with studies by Schoder and colleagues [28] and Zanation and colleagues [29], where management was altered in 18.0% and 21.6% of the patients, respectively. By detection of synchronous or metastatic disease, information provided by PET/CT led to changes in planned procedures or sparing of previously planned procedure and also helped guide biopsy to metabolically active areas in the larynx [30]. However, it is still unclear how PET/CT compares with the combination of CT, MRI, and/or PET scan as it is currently used in some institutions.

PET/CT in post-treatment evaluation

While PET/CT has found increased use in the pretreatment period, its greatest utility may be in the setting of detecting recurrent cancer after radiation therapy and/or surgery, where the resultant anatomic changes are difficult to characterize by traditional imaging modalities (CT, MRI) alone. PET/CT already has a track record of high sensitivity and specificity in detection of recurrences of head and neck cancers in general. One of the few studies looking specifically at laryngeal cancer surveillance demonstrated a sensitivity of 93.75% and specificity of 91.67% in determining recurrence when the standardized uptake value threshold was set at 3.35 [31]. However, PET/CT does have low but measurable false-positive rates due to the increased metabolic activity in areas of infection or chronic inflammation.

Metastatic work-up

In the absence of advanced laryngeal carcinoma and cervical metastasis, distant spread of tumor is rare. Spector and colleagues [32] reviewed 1667 patients with primary laryngeal carcinoma and found an overall metastasis incidence of 3.6%, 4.4%, and 14.2% for supraglottic, glottic, and subglottic tumors respectively. The incidence of distant metastasis for supraglottic tumors correlated with the presence of cervical metastasis while the incidence for glottic tumors correlated with T-stage and subglottic tumors demonstrated no relationship to TNM staging. A study of 202 supraglottic and 270 glottic tumors out of Pittsburgh had a higher incidence of distant metastasis overall but still relatively low compared with other cancers—supraglottic (11%), glottic (7%) [33–35].

Routine work-up for metastatic disease in laryngeal carcinoma is not universally advocated and often institution dependent. Lung, followed by liver, are the most frequent sites of distant metastasis and as such chest radiographs and laboratory investigation of liver function tests (LFTs) with possible liver ultrasonography has been the minimal standard at several institutions [3]. Patients with an abnormal chest x-ray (CXR) and those with advanced disease or high clinical suspicion may warrant CT of the chest and abdomen. Recently, the practice of obtaining a pretreatment PET/CT on patients with advanced stage laryngeal carcinomas has become more frequent, but the jury is still out on routine use of PET/CT scan for pretreatment work-up of laryngeal malignancies.

Routine preoperative laboratory tests are indicated in patients who are likely to receive treatment—either surgery or chemoradiation. Chemistry to include BUN (blood urea nitrogen), creatinine, and LFT and CBC (complete blood count) are typically required regardless of treatment plan. Elevated calcium or alkaline phosphatase may be a sign of metastatic disease. In addition, pre-albumin, albumin, and transferrin may be useful to assess the patient's nutritional status. Thyroid function evaluation is necessary in case of history of previous radiation treatment/thyroid surgery.

Operative assessment

Despite an adequate examination in the office including laryngoscopy and tumor mapping, most patients with laryngeal carcinoma require a trip to the operating room for formal endoscopic examination and biopsy under anesthesia.

Direct laryngoscopy

Preoperative discussion of the airway between the surgeon and the anesthesiologist, and formulation of a primary plan and backup plans to secure the airway is critical in the operative assessment. In the event of a large supraglottic tumor or anterior larynx, the Hollinger anterior commisure laryngoscope may be used to gain access to the airway. Once the airway is secured, the Hollinger laryngoscope may also be used for the initial survey of laryngeal structures. Depending on the site of lesion, critical assessment of the lesion may only be possible under apneic conditions. As such, communication with competent anesthesiologists is critical.

Once the patient has been intubated, the selection of laryngoscope is largely dependent on surgeon preference and on the patient's anatomy. A variety of scopes exist, each with their own pros and cons and they are often used in combination. The Dedo laryngoscope can be considered the workhorse scope. It has a larger caliber compared with the Hollinger and allows for greater distention of soft tissues and the larger proximal inlet facilitates the use of multiple instruments including rigid telescopes and also allows for binocular vision using the microscope. The Lindholm laryngoscope is a vallecular scope and has a large caliber distal opening, which allows for a more global view of the larynx and surrounding structures as well as facilitating the simultaneous use of instruments and telescopes. It is preferable to map the lesion after completing the endoscopic assessment for synchronous or metachronous lesions. This ensures that blood from the tumor and the biopsy sites will not obscure visualization during surveillance endoscopy.

Is panendoscopy still indicated?

Panendoscopy including laryngoscopy, esophagoscopy, and bronchoscopy has been the standard for many years. However, with improved preoperative imaging some centers do not consider panendoscopy a standard part of the diagnostic work-up. Others have advocated symptom-directed endoscopies based on the fact that most second primaries are revealed by their specific symptoms [36]. Supporters of continued panendoscopy argue that while the number of simultaneous second primary tumors identified at endoscopy may be relative low, the significance of a positive finding is often critical to the individual. Furthermore, lesions identified at endoscopy may be found at an earlier stage and are more amenable to cure when the patient is asymptomatic and the lesion undetectable radiographically.

Assessment of the larynx should include both piriform sinuses and the postcricoid area. It is often useful to place the patient in suspension and to use the 0°, 30°, and 70° telescopes. The use of a rigid telescope allows for magnification and superior visualization of the subglottis, anterior commisure, and the ventricle—all areas difficult to adequately visualize in the clinic. The laryngeal probe permits assessment of extension into the ventricle in the event that telescopes are not used. While vocal fold mobility is best assessed in the office with indirect mirror or fiber-optic examination, palpation of the vocal process in the operating room can help distinguish true vocal fold paralysis from arytenoid fixation. This is critical not only for staging but also to evaluate the cricoarytenoid unit whose function is necessary for many laryngeal conservation procedures. The extent of the laryngeal lesion should be either photographed or mapped on a standardized schematic of the larynx (Fig. 4).

Biopsy

Although squamous cell carcinoma accounts for the great majority of laryngeal malignancies, a biopsy-proven pathologic diagnosis of a primary site is required before proceeding to definitive management. The gross appearance of other benign lesions such as laryngeal tuberculosis, Wegener's granulomatosis, sarcoidosis, and fungal laryngitis can be mistaken for advanced laryngeal carcinoma.

To prove the presence of invasive carcinoma, the biopsy should be deep enough to reach viable tumor and stroma or muscle. Biopsy sites should include the obvious lesion of interest and any suspicious lesions on the contralateral arytenoid, anterior commisure, or interarytenoid area because of the ramifications of positive biopsies in these areas for conservation laryngeal surgery. If the lesion is small or amenable to resection without engendering undue complications, such as notching of the vocal cord or blunting of the anterior commisure, it should be completely excised to create a satisfactory specimen. In any event, small superficial lesions require a small cuff of normal-appearing submucosa to ascertain the depth of invasion, while larger lesions should be adequately sampled with biopsy forceps to measure invasion below the basement membrane. In the context of continued clinical suspicion, repeat biopsies are warranted and are often needed to diagnose carcinoma in situ or microinvasion in small lesions originally read as benign or dysplastic.

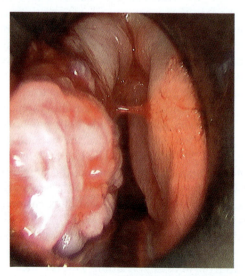

Fig. 4. Operative endoscopy of T3 supraglottic SCCA.

Newer/novel diagnostic modalities

Various new techniques have been introduced to improve the diagnostic accuracy of microlaryngoscopy. Autofluorescence diagnosis is based on the ability of oxidized flavin mononucleotide (FMN) in normal cells to emit green fluorescence when exposed to blue light. Neoplastic cells can be distinguished by their significantly lower levels of FMN and consequently do not fluoresce to the same degree. Initial studies have shown some promise with increased accuracy and a tendency toward earlier detection of early laryngeal cancers [37,38]. Less data are available for contact endoscopy in which the laryngeal mucosa is stained with 1% methylene blue and examined under special endoscopes with ×60 to ×150 magnification. The staining and magnification allows visualization of the cells, nuclei, and cytoplasm of laryngeal mucosa and their different grades of abnormality [39]. However, this technique requires specialized instrumentation and also experience in pathologic diagnosis of laryngeal lesions, which is outside the scope of training received by most head and neck surgeons.

Tumor thickness as a prognosticator

Tumor thickness is a well-established prognostic indicator in melanoma and most recently has found use in carcinoma of the oral cavity and oropharynx. More recently, tumor thickness has been indirectly correlated with prognosis in laryngeal cancer. A retrospective study of 111 T1-3 laryngeal cancer patients treated with surgery found tumor thickness was significantly related to T, N, and clinical stage as well as pathologic cervical lymph node metastasis, cartilage invasion, microscopic appearance, perineural invasion, and lymphatic invasion [40]. Dadas and colleagues [41] proved the feasibility of intraoperative assessment of tumor thickness in laryngeal cancer patients by frozen section analysis. Although frozen sections are not routinely performed to assess tumor thickness, frozen section analysis is commonly used to ensure adequacy of the specimen for repeat endoscopy. Frozen section results may also alert the pathologist to certain lesions that require immediate or special handling such as preparation for electron microscopy [42]. However, these studies do not clarify whether the depth of invasion on histology will assist the clinician in formulating the treatment plan.

Molecular diagnosis

The reader is directed to the article by Loyo and Pai on "The Molecular Genetics of Laryngeal Cancer" in this issue for a more in-depth review of this topic. Squamous cell carcinoma (SCC) accounts for approximately 95% of all laryngeal malignancies. SCC of the head and neck arises from premalignant progenitors followed by growth of clonal populations associated with cumulative genetic alterations and phenotypic progression to invasive malignancy. These genetic changes lead to inactivation of multiple tumor suppressor genes and activation of proto-oncogenes such as p53, cyclin D1, epidermal growth factor receptor (EGFR), and others [43–45]. Epigenetic changes have also been linked to the pathophysiology of head and neck SCC.

One avenue for improved detection of minimal disease in surgical margins has been the study of molecular alterations in pathologically negative tumor margins. The presence and clinical implication of these alterations have been studied in large multicenter trials. The tumor suppressor gene, p53, has emerged as a potential marker for the development of local recurrence. Brennan and colleagues [46], in a study of 25 patients with microscopic negative surgical margins, found that 5 of 13 patients with p53 mutations detected in the original specimen went on to develop local recurrences. None of the 12 patients without detectable p53 mutations developed local recurrence of their tumors during the course of the study. These results have been replicated by others as well [47].

eIF4E, a eukaryotic protein synthesis initiation factor elevated in almost all head and neck squamous cell cancers, has been reported to be an even more sensitive prognostic indicator for local recurrences compared with p53. Using immunohistochemical techniques, Nathan and colleagues [48] demonstrated statistically significant differences in local recurrence rates and disease-free survival intervals between eIF4E-positive and eIF4E-negative margins. eIF4E-positive patients had a 6.5-fold relative risk of developing local recurrences compared with eIF4E-negative patients.

However, despite our improved understanding of the molecular basis of head and neck cancer, these advances have yet to offer efficacious clinically relevant treatments. Smoking cessation for those at risk for the development of head and neck cancers including laryngeal cancer remains the most effective means of prevention.

Staging

The last modification of the AJCC TNM staging protocol occurred in 2002 (Appendix). Although this staging provides prognostic information, it does not stratify the patients into the various treatment modalities to assist the clinicians. To this end, the American Society of Clinical Oncology formed a multidisciplinary Expert Panel to review the current literature available through November of 2005 [49]. One finding was the lack of randomized prospective trials to direct evidence-based treatment algorithms. Regardless, the report did recommend that T1 and T2 laryngeal cancer should be treated with the intent to preserve the laryngeal function with a single modality. For most T3 and T4 without extensive cartilage invasion, an organ-preservation modality is an appropriate and standard treatment option. However, no organ-conservation modality offered a survival advantage in comparison to total laryngectomy.

Histology

Squamous cell carcinoma constitutes the overwhelming majority of laryngeal malignancies: 90% to 95%. One note about the histology of laryngeal SCCA is that the grade of the carcinoma is not predictive of prognosis, unlike SCCA in some of the other areas of the head and neck. There are recent reports that the depth of invasion may correlate with its aggressive behavior, but these findings have yet to be corroborated.

Several clinical dilemmas present themselves when leukoplakia is diagnosed with dysplasia. First, histologic grading must assess whether the dysplasia is severe or, even worse, carcinoma in situ (CIS) or Tis. The distinction between severe dysplasia and CIS is controversial and pathologist-dependent. Frequently, repeat biopsies may be necessary to clarify these subjective findings and to rule out any evidence of invasive carcinoma. There have been reports that aneuploidy has been associated with recurrence and progression to carcinoma, but there are currently no accepted objective tests for these subtypes that may require more aggressive management. For patients with severe dysplasia, it is not uncommon for them to undergo multiple excisional surgeries or laser ablations with close follow-up, and still develop frank carcinoma.

An abbreviated differential diagnosis for malignant laryngeal tumors consists of basaloid squamous cell carcinoma, verrucous carcinoma, spindle cell carcinoma, glandular carcinomas (adenocarcinoma not otherwise specified [NOS], adenoid cystic, mucoepidermoid), and sarcomas (chondrosarcoma and liposarcoma). Among the glandular tumors, adenocarcinoma NOS is most common, while chondrosarcoma, which typically presents at the posterior lamina of the cricoid, is more frequently seen than liposarcoma. In general, most of these uncommon laryngeal malignancies require surgery as part of the treatment modality. Within the SCCA spectrum, basaloid squamous cell carcinoma represents a more aggressive pathology that presents with much more advanced disease, while verrucous carcinoma behaves like a low-grade tumor with a very low tendency to metastasize to the draining lymph node. However, because of reports of "anaplastic transformation" following radiotherapy, verrucous carcinomas are traditionally treated with surgery without an elective neck dissection.

Follow-up

Although laryngeal cancer patients are treated by a multidisciplinary team, the surgeon should play the leadership role during the follow-up period. Most recurrences occur in the first 2 years after primary treatment, so a complete otolaryngologic history and examination is mandatory within this time frame. The clinical visits are typically spaced every 4 to 6 weeks the first year and every 8 to 12 weeks the second year. Annual visit can be done after the fifth year. There are no serum markers or radiographic tests that are recommended at this point. PET/CT scan showed some early promise, but it has yet to be validated for surveillance purposes.

Appendix

TNM staging of laryngeal carcinoma

Primary tumor (T)
>   TX: Primary tumor cannot be assessed
>   T0: No evidence of primary tumor
>   Tis: Carcinoma in situ

Supraglottis
>   T1: Tumor limited to one subsite* of supraglottis with normal vocal cord mobility
>   T2: Tumor invades mucosa of more than one adjacent subsite* of supraglottis or glottis or region outside the supraglottis (eg, mucosa of base of tongue, vallecula, or medial wall of pyriform sinus) without fixation of the larynx
>   T3: Tumor limited to larynx with vocal cord fixation and/or invades any of the following: postcricoid area, pre-epiglottic tissues, paraglottic space, and/or minor thyroid cartilage erosion (eg, inner cortex)
>   T4a: Tumor invades through the thyroid cartilage, and/or invades tissues beyond the larynx (eg, trachea, soft tissues of the neck including deep extrinsic muscle of the tongue, strap muscles, thyroid, or esophagus)
>   T4b: Tumor invades prevertebral space, encases carotid artery, or invades mediastinal structures
>>   Subsites include the following:
>>   Ventricular bands (false cords)
>>   Arytenoids
>>   Suprahyoid epiglottis
>>   Infrahyoid epiglottis
>>   Aryepiglottic folds (laryngeal aspect)

[Note: Supraglottis involves many individual subsites. Relapse-free survival may differ by subsite and by T and N groupings within stage.]

Glottis
>   T1: Tumor limited to the vocal cord(s), which may involve anterior or posterior commissure, with normal mobility
>>   T1a: Tumor limited to one vocal cord
>>   T1b: Tumor involves both vocal cords
>   T2: Tumor extends to supraglottis and/or subglottis and/or with impaired vocal cord mobility
>   T3: Tumor limited to the larynx with vocal cord fixation and/or invades paraglottic space, and/or minor thyroid cartilage erosion (eg, inner cortex)

T4a: Tumor invades through the thyroid cartilage and/or invades tissues beyond the larynx (eg, trachea, soft tissues of neck, including deep extrinsic muscle of the tongue, strap muscles, thyroid, or esophagus)

T4b: Tumor invades prevertebral space, encases carotid artery, or invades mediastinal structures

[Note: Glottic presentation may vary by volume of tumor, anatomic region involved, and the presence or absence of normal cord mobility. Relapse-free survival may differ by these and other factors in addition to T and N subgroupings within the stage.]

Subglottis

T1: Tumor limited to the subglottis

T2: Tumor extends to vocal cord(s) with normal or impaired mobility

T3: Tumor limited to larynx with vocal cord fixation

T4a: Tumor invades cricoid or thyroid cartilage and/or invades tissues beyond the larynx (eg, trachea, soft tissues of neck, including deep extrinsic muscles of the tongue, strap muscles, thyroid, or esophagus)

T4b: Tumor invades prevertebral space, encases carotid artery, or invades mediastinal structures

Regional lymph nodes (N)

NX: Regional lymph nodes cannot be assessed

N0: No regional lymph node metastasis

N1: Metastasis in a single ipsilateral lymph node 3 cm or smaller in greatest dimension

N2: Metastasis in a single ipsilateral lymph node larger than 3 cm but 6 cm or smaller in greatest dimension, or in multiple ipsilateral lymph nodes 6 cm or smaller in greatest dimension, or in bilateral or contralateral lymph nodes 6 cm or smaller in greatest dimension

N2a: Metastasis in a single ipsilateral lymph node larger than 3 cm but 6 cm or smaller in greatest dimension

N2b: Metastasis in multiple ipsilateral lymph nodes 6 cm or smaller in greatest dimension

N2c: Metastasis in bilateral or contralateral lymph nodes 6 cm or smaller in greatest dimension

N3: Metastasis in a lymph node larger than 6 cm in greatest dimension

In clinical evaluation, the actual size of the nodal mass should be measured, and allowance should be made for intervening soft tissues. Most masses larger than 3 cm in diameter are not single nodes but confluent nodes or tumors in soft tissues of the neck. There are three stages of clinically positive nodes: N1, N2, and N3. The use of subgroups a, b, and c is not required but recommended. Midline nodes are considered homolateral nodes.

Distant metastasis (M)
  MX: Distant metastasis cannot be assessed
  M0: No distant metastasis
  M1: Distant metastasis
AJCC Stage Groupings
  Stage 0
    Tis, N0, M0
  Stage I
    T1, N0, M0
  Stage II
    T2, N0, M0
  Stage III
    T3, N0, M0
    T1, N1, M0
    T2, N1, M0
    T3, N1, M0
  Stage IVA
    T4a, N0, M0
    T4a, N1, M0
    T1, N2, M0
    T2, N2, M0
    T3, N2, M0
    T4a, N2, M0
  Stage IVB
    T4b, any N, M0
    Any T, N3, M0
  Stage IVC
    Any T, any N, M1

Evaluation of treatment outcome can be reported in various ways: locoregional control, disease-free survival, determinate survival, and overall survival at 2 to 5 years. Preservation of voice is an important parameter to evaluate. Outcome should be reported after initial surgery, initial radiation, planned combined treatment, or surgical salvage of radiation failures. Primary source material should be consulted to review these differences.

Because of clinical problems related to smoking and alcohol use in this population, many patients succumb to intercurrent illness rather than to the primary cancer. Direct comparison of results of radiation versus surgery is complicated. Surgical studies can report outcome based on pathologic staging, whereas radiation studies must report on clinical staging, with the obvious problem of understaging in patients treated with radiation, particularly in the neck. In addition, radiation alone is often recommended for patients with poor performance status, which leads to less favorable results.

From American Joint Committee on Cancer: AJCC Cancer Staging Manual. Larynx. 6th ed. New York, NY: Springer; 2002. p. 47–57.

References

[1] American Cancer Society. Cancer facts and figures. 2007. American Cancer Society; 2007. Available at: http://www.cancer.org/docroot/STT/stt_0_2007.asp?sitearea = STT&level = 1.

[2] McNeil BJ, Weichselbaum R, Pauker SG. Speech and survival: tradeoffs between quality and quantity of life in laryngeal cancer. N Engl J Med 1981;305(17):982–7.

[3] Marioni G, Marchese-Ragona R, Cartei G, et al. Current opinion in diagnosis and treatment of laryngeal carcinoma. Cancer Treat Rev 2006;32(7):504–15.

[4] Sadler TW. Head and neck. In: Coryell P, editor. Langman's medical embryology. Baltimore (MD): Lippincott Williams and Wilkins; 1995. p. 312–46.

[5] Beitler JJ, Mahadevia PS, Silver CE, et al. New barriers to ventricular invasion in paraglottic laryngeal cancer. Cancer 1994;73(10):2648–52.

[6] Pressman J, Dowdy A, Libby R, et al. Further studies upon the submucosal compartments and lymphatics of the larynx by the injection of dyes and radioisotopes. Ann Otol Rhinol Laryngol 1956;65(4):963–80.

[7] Jemal A, Tiwari RC, Murray T, et al. Cancer statistics, 2004. CA Cancer J Clin 2004;54(1): 8–29.

[8] Thekdi AA, Ferris RL. Diagnostic assessment of laryngeal cancer. Otolaryngol Clin North Am 2002;35(5):953–69, v.

[9] Sadri M, McMahon J, Parker A. Laryngeal dysplasia: aetiology and molecular biology. J Laryngol Otol 2006;120(3):170–7.

[10] Talamini R, Bosetti C, La Vecchia C, et al. Combined effect of tobacco and alcohol on laryngeal cancer risk: a case-control study. Cancer Causes Control 2002;13(10): 957–64.

[11] Tuyns AJ, Esteve J, Raymond L, et al. Cancer of the larynx/hypopharynx, tobacco and alcohol: IARC international case-control study in Turin and Varese (Italy), Zaragoza and Navarra (Spain), Geneva (Switzerland) and Calvados (France). Int J Cancer 1988;41(4): 483–91.

[12] Bosetti C, Garavello W, Gallus S, et al. Effects of smoking cessation on the risk of laryngeal cancer: an overview of published studies. Oral Oncol 2006;42(9):866–72.

[13] Muscat JE, Wynder EL. Tobacco, alcohol, asbestos, and occupational risk factors for laryngeal cancer. Cancer 1992;69(9):2244–51.

[14] El Serag HB, Hepworth EJ, Lee P, et al. Gastroesophageal reflux disease is a risk factor for laryngeal and pharyngeal cancer. Am J Gastroenterol 2001;96(7):2013–8.

[15] Capone RB, Pai SI, Koch WM, et al. Detection and quantitation of human papillomavirus (HPV) DNA in the sera of patients with HPV-associated head and neck squamous cell carcinoma. Clin Cancer Res 2000;6(11):4171–5.

[16] Gillison ML, Koch WM, Capone RB, et al. Evidence for a causal association between human papillomavirus and a subset of head and neck cancers. J Natl Cancer Inst 2000; 92(9):709–20.

[17] Breau RL, Suen JY. Management of the N(0) neck. Otolaryngol Clin North Am 1998;31(4): 657–69.

[18] Million RR, Cassisi NJ. Radical irradiation for carcinoma of the pyriform sinus. Laryngoscope 1981;91(3):439–50.

[19] Postma GN, Bach KK, Belafsky PC, et al. The role of transnasal esophagoscopy in head and neck oncology. Laryngoscope 2002;112(12):2242–3.

[20] Yousem DM, Gad K, Tufano RP. Resectability issues with head and neck cancer. AJNR Am J Neuroradiol 2006;27(10):2024–36.

[21] Becker M, Zbaren P, Laeng H, et al. Neoplastic invasion of the laryngeal cartilage: comparison of MR imaging and CT with histopathologic correlation. Radiology 1995;194(3): 661–9.

[22] Becker M, Zbaren P, Delavelle J, et al. Neoplastic invasion of the laryngeal cartilage: reassessment of criteria for diagnosis at CT. Radiology 1997;203(2):521–32.

[23] Zbaren P, Becker M, Lang H. Pretherapeutic staging of hypopharyngeal carcinoma. Clinical findings, computed tomography, and magnetic resonance imaging compared with histopathologic evaluation. Arch Otolaryngol Head Neck Surg 1997;123(9):908–13.

[24] Sessions RB, Picken CA. Malignant cervical adenopathy. In: Cummings CW, Fredrickson JM, Harker LA, et al, editors. Otolaryngology-Head and Neck Surgery. St. Louis (MO): Mosby-Year Book; 1988. p. 737–57.

[25] Yousem DM, Hatabu H, Hurst RW, et al. Carotid artery invasion by head and neck masses: prediction with MR imaging. Radiology 1995;195(3):715–20.

[26] Loevner LA, Ott IL, Yousem DM, et al. Neoplastic fixation to the prevertebral compartment by squamous cell carcinoma of the head and neck. AJR Am J Roentgenol 1998;170(5): 1389–94.

[27] Fleming AJ Jr, Smith SP Jr, Paul CM, et al. Impact of [18F]-2-fluorodeoxyglucose-positron emission tomography/computed tomography on previously untreated head and neck cancer patients. Laryngoscope 2007;117(7):1173–9.

[28] Schoder H, Yeung HW, Gonen M, et al. Head and neck cancer: clinical usefulness and accuracy of PET/CT image fusion. Radiology 2004;231(1):65–72.

[29] Zanation AM, Sutton DK, Couch ME, et al. Use, accuracy, and implications for patient management of [18F]-2-fluorodeoxyglucose-positron emission/computerized tomography for head and neck tumors. Laryngoscope 2005;115(7):1186–90.

[30] Gordin A, Daitzchman M, Doweck I, et al. Fluorodeoxyglucose-positron emission tomography/computed tomography imaging in patients with carcinoma of the larynx: diagnostic accuracy and impact on clinical management. Laryngoscope 2006;116(2): 273–8.

[31] Oe A, Kawabe J, Torii K, et al. Detection of local residual tumor after laryngeal cancer treatment using FDG-PET. Ann Nucl Med 2007;21(1):9–13.

[32] Spector GJ. Distant metastases from laryngeal and hypopharyngeal cancer. ORL J Otorhinolaryngol Relat Spec 2001;63(4):224–8.

[33] Johnson JT. Carcinoma of the larynx: selective approach to the management of cervical lymphatics. Ear Nose Throat J 1994;73(5):303–5.

[34] Kryj M, Maciejewski B, Withers HR, et al. Incidence and kinetics of distant metastases in patients with operable breast cancer. Neoplasma 1997;44(1):3–11.

[35] Shah H, Anker CJ, Bogart J, et al. Brain: the common site of relapse in patients with pancoast or superior sulcus tumors. J Thorac Oncol 2006;1(9):1020–2.

[36] Benninger MS, Shariff A, Blazoff K. Symptom-directed selective endoscopy: long-term efficacy. Arch Otolaryngol Head Neck Surg 2001;127(7):770–3.

[37] Chissov VI, Sokolov VV, Filonenko EV, et al. (Clinical fluorescent diagnosis of tumors using photosensitizer photogem). Khirurgiia (Mosk) 1995;(5):37–41 [in Russian].

[38] Harries ML, Lam S, MacAulay C, et al. Diagnostic imaging of the larynx: autofluorescence of laryngeal tumours using the helium-cadmium laser. J Laryngol Otol 1995;109(2):108–10.

[39] Arens C, Malzahn K, Dias O, et al. (Endoscopic imaging techniques in the diagnosis of laryngeal carcinoma and its precursor lesions). Laryngorhinootologie 1999;78(12):685–91 [in German].

[40] Yilmaz T, Gedikoglu G, Gursel B. The relationship between tumor thickness and clinical and histopathologic parameters in cancer of the larynx. Otolaryngol Head Neck Surg 2003;129(3):192–8.

[41] Dadas B, Basak T, Ozdemir T, et al. Reliability of frozen section in determining tumor thickness intraoperatively in laryngeal cancer. Laryngoscope 2000;110(12):2070–3.

[42] Barney PL. Histopathologic problems and frozen section diagnosis in diseases of the larynx. Otolaryngol Clin North Am 1970;3(3):493–515.

[43] Perez-Ordonez B, Beauchemin M, Jordan RC. Molecular biology of squamous cell carcinoma of the head and neck. J Clin Pathol 2006;59(5):445–53.

[44] Fearon ER, Vogelstein B. A genetic model for colorectal tumorigenesis. Cell 1990;61(5): 759–67.

[45] Knudson AG Jr. Mutation and cancer: statistical study of retinoblastoma. Proc Natl Acad Sci U S A 1971;68(4):820–3.

[46] Brennan JA, Mao L, Hruban RH, et al. Molecular assessment of histopathological staging in squamous-cell carcinoma of the head and neck. N Engl J Med 1995;332(7):429–35.

[47] van Houten VM, Leemans CR, Kummer JA, et al. Molecular diagnosis of surgical margins and local recurrence in head and neck cancer patients: a prospective study. Clin Cancer Res 2004;10(11):3614–20.

[48] Nathan CO, Amirghahri N, Rice C, et al. Molecular analysis of surgical margins in head and neck squamous cell carcinoma patients. Laryngoscope 2002;112(12):2129–40.

[49] Pfister DG, Laurie SA, Weinstein GS, et al. American Society of Clinical Oncology clinical practice guideline for the use of larynx—preservation strategies in the treatment of laryngeal cancer. J Clin Oncol 2006;24(22):3693–704.

ELSEVIER
SAUNDERS

Otolaryngol Clin N Am
41 (2008) 697–713

OTOLARYNGOLOGIC
CLINICS
OF NORTH AMERICA

Radiologic Evaluation of Larynx Cancer

Ari M. Blitz, MD*, Nafi Aygun, MD

*Division of Neuroradiology, The Russell H. Morgan Department of Radiology and
Radiological Science, Johns Hopkins University, 600 North Wolfe Street, Phipps B-100,
Baltimore, MD 21287, USA*

Clinical examination (including endoscopy and biopsy) of the larynx allows an accurate assessment of superficial spread of neoplasm. Pathologic involvement of the deep spaces of the larynx is greatly underestimated by the clinical examination, however. Imaging, conversely, fails to detect superficial mucosal disease and tends to overestimate the deep extent of tumor. The combination of information from cross-sectional imaging when taken together with information gleaned from clinical examination provides the most accurate pretherapeutic staging of laryngeal neoplasm. For this reason, close collaboration with a radiologist skilled in the performance and interpretation of imaging of the head and neck is especially vital to direct successful therapy of patients who have neoplasm of the larynx.

Imaging anatomy of the larynx

The larynx is a hollow tube lined by mucosa and adapted for protection of the airway and phonation. The cartilaginous scaffolding of the larynx is composed of the thyroid, cricoid, and arytenoid cartilages surrounded by connective and muscular tissue that form its walls. Superiorly, the epiglottis demarcates the boundary with the pharynx. Inferiorly, the larynx extends to the lower margin of the cricoid. Laryngeal anatomy is divided into supraglottic, glottic, and subglottic regions (Fig. 1).

Supraglottis

The supraglottic larynx extends from the epiglottis and laryngeal surface of the aryepiglottic folds superiorly through the laryngeal ventricle

---

* Corresponding author. The Johns Hopkins Medical Institution, 600 North Wolfe Street, Phipps B-100, Baltimore, MD 21287.

E-mail address: ablitz1@jhmi.edu (A.M. Blitz).

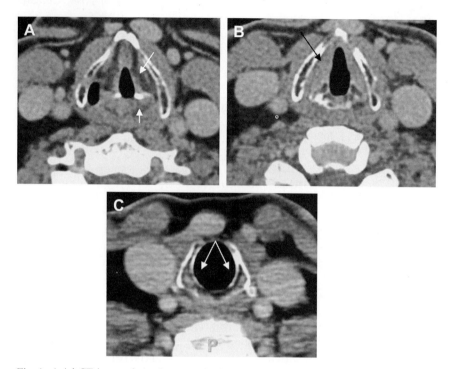

Fig. 1. Axial CT images from the supraglottic (*A*), glottic (*B*), and subglottic (*C*) levels. (*A*) Note that submucosal fat (*long arrow*) is seen in the supraglottic level. The short arrow points to the arytenoid cartilage. (*B*) No submucosal fat is apparent at the level of glottis because of the thyroarytenoid muscle (*arrow*). (*C*) There is no submucosal tissue in the subglottis at the level of the cricoid ring so that the air column abuts the cartilage (*arrows*).

inferiorly. The supraglottic larynx is delimited inferiorly by the superior surface of the true vocal cords. On cross-sectional imaging, the false vocal folds are easily discriminated from the true cords by submucosal presence of fat in the former. The pre-epiglottic space is filled with fat tissue (Fig. 2C). Robust lymphatic drainage to the high deep cervical chain contributes to the higher incidence of nodal metastasis at the time of diagnosis of lesions in this region.

Glottis

The vocal folds (true vocal cords) and anterior and posterior commissures comprise the glottis (Fig. 2A, B). Superiorly, the glottis is bounded by the supraglottic larynx; inferiorly, it is bounded by the subglottic larynx. Radiologically, the vocal folds are easily distinguished from the false vocal cords by the presence of submucosal soft tissue density attributable to the vocalis muscle. Lymphatic drainage from the glottis itself is sparse, and nodal metastasis from lesions in this region is rare.

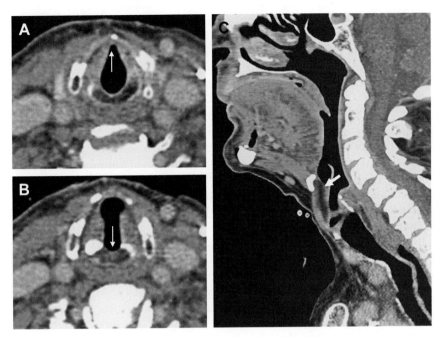

Fig. 2. Axial CT image through the glottis. Arrows point to the anterior commissure (*A*) and the posterior commissure. (*B*) Note lack of submucosal tissue in these regions. (*C*) Sagittal CT shows the pre-epiglottic space (*arrow*) as a dark area because of low x-ray attenuation of fat.

Subglottis

The subglottis extends from the inferior surface of the vocal fold to the inferior extent of the cricoid cartilage and is difficult to visualize in the office. The endoluminal contour of the subglottis is normally smooth (see Fig. 1C). The presence of subglottic soft tissue should raise suspicion of neoplastic invasion. Lymphatic drainage from the subglottis is sparse, and nodal metastasis from lesions in this region is rare.

Choosing modality of imaging

CT versus MRI

State-of-the-art multichannel CT affords high spatial resolution images that can be reformatted in any desired plane, essentially negating the traditional advantage of MRI because of its multiplanar capability. Superior contrast resolution and multiparametric imaging (eg, T1-weighted, T2-weighted) remain significant advantages of MRI.

CT evaluation is much faster than MRI, substantially reducing or eliminating artifacts of movement attributable to breathing, swallowing, or coughing. MRI is more resource-intensive and less available than CT.

Overall, the staging accuracy of MRI in laryngeal cancer is slightly higher, largely because of more accurate assessment of cartilage involvement and paraglottic pre-epiglottic extension of tumor. CT is still more commonly used compared with MRI for initial staging of laryngeal cancer because of practical advantages, such as cost, speed, and availability.

Positron emission tomography–CT

Studies with sufficiently large numbers of patients investigating the role of positron emission tomography (PET)–CT in staging of laryngeal cancer are lacking. Recent reports suggest that PET evaluation of head and neck cancers may not present sufficient sensitivity or specificity to justify its routine use at the time of initial diagnosis [1], whereas others have reported that it significantly altered treatment in a substantial number of patients [2]. Given the intrinsic limitation of spatial resolution of PET examination and its inability to assess lesions of small volume adequately, it would be unrealistic to expect that PET would improve T-staging of laryngeal cancer compared with clinical examination and CT or MRI. The accuracy of N-staging by PET is superior to other methods; however, currently, the negative predictive value of PET in nodal metastasis assessment is not sufficiently high to justify a change in treatment. PET has a distinct advantage compared with CT or MRI for detection of distant metastasis and should be routinely performed in patients with high risk for distant metastasis or when the primary site of neoplasm is unknown [3,4]. It is possible that future development of more specific tracers or other improvements in technology may remedy some of these limitations. The role of PET-CT in posttreatment follow-up is well established by comparison, and PET-CT at the time of diagnosis may still provide a useful baseline for further management in some cases. Furthermore, PET imaging may be used to facilitate radiotherapy planning, which may provide sufficient justification for performing PET-CT at the time of initial imaging.

Malignant lesions of the larynx and staging

Supraglottis

The supraglottis is divided for the purposes of staging into several subsites: suprahyoid epiglottis, infrahyoid epiglottis, laryngeal surface of aryepiglottic folds, arytenoids, and false vocal cords. Nodal metastasis to levels II to IV is frequently seen. Essential imaging features include vocal cord fixation; tumor volume; and pre-epiglottic, paraglottic, and transglottic spread of disease.

T1: Tumor is confined to the site of origin, involving one supraglottic subsite. There is normal vocal cord mobility.

T2: Tumor extends to adjacent portions of the supraglottis or glottis (or adjacent extralaryngeal site, such as mucosa of the tongue base, vallecula, or medial wall of the piriform sinus). There is normal vocal cord mobility.

T3: There is vocal cord fixation or involvement of the pre-epiglottic space, paraglottic space, or inner cortex of the cartilages.

T4:

> T4a: Tumor invades through the thyroid cartilage or invades tissues beyond the larynx.
>
> T4b: Tumor invades the prevertebral space, encases the carotid artery, or invades mediastinal structures.

Glottis

T1: Tumor is confined to the vocal fold. The vocal fold retains normal mobility.

> T1a: Involvement of a single vocal fold
>
> T1b: Involvement of both vocal folds

T2: Tumor extends superiorly into the supraglottis or inferiorly into the subglottic region, or vocal cord mobility is altered.

T3: The vocal cords are fixed; however, tumor is confined to the larynx. The paraglottic space and the inner cortex of the cartilages may be involved,

T4:

> T4a: Tumor invades through the thyroid cartilage or invades tissues beyond the larynx.
>
> T4b: Tumor invades the prevertebral space, encases the carotid artery, or invades mediastinal structures.

Subglottic larynx

An isolated subglottic neoplasm is uncommon. Nodal drainage from this region includes level IV and level VI lymph nodes and the upper mediastinal lymph nodes.

T1: Tumor is confined to the subglottis.

T2: Tumor extends to the vocal folds.

T3: There is vocal cord fixation, but tumor remains confined to the larynx.

T4:

> T4a: Tumor invades through the thyroid cartilage or invades tissues beyond the larynx.
>
> T4b: Tumor invades the prevertebral space, encases the carotid artery, or invades mediastinal structures.

Pre-epiglottic and paraglottic space invasion

The pre-epiglottic space is situated between the epiglottis anteriorly and the hyoid bone, thyrohyoid membrane, and thyroid cartilage anteriorly. The pre-epiglottic space is readily identified on noncontrast T1-weighted MRI or

CT, particularly in the sagittal plane, because of its largely fatty contents. On either side, the pre-epiglottic space is continuous with the paraglottic space (also known as the paralaryngeal space). The paraglottic space spans between the thyrohyoid membrane, thyroid and cricoid cartilages laterally and between the false and true vocal cords and the elastic cone medially. It contains fat at the level of the false vocal cords. This can be easily identified on axial and sagittal noncontrast T1-weighted MRI and CT, because fat tissue has unique imaging features. Invasion of the pre-epiglottic fat by glottic or supraglottic carcinomas is difficult to appreciate on clinical examination but is often readily appreciated by the head and neck radiologist as replacement of the normal fat on CT or MRI (Figs. 3–5) [5]. Likewise, imaging detection of paraglottic space involvement is reliable.

Anterior and posterior commissures

Between the attachment sites of the vocal cords to the thyroid cartilage is a "bare" area, wherein the laryngeal mucosa abuts the thyroid cartilage. This is known as the anterior commissure. The mucosa covering the posterior wall of the glottis between the arytenoid cartilages is known as the posterior commissure. There is no submucosal tissue present in the anterior and

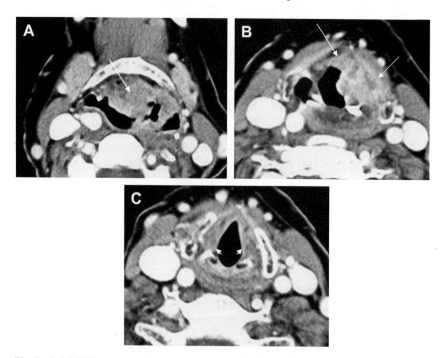

Fig. 3. Axial CT images through the supraglottis (*A*, *B*) and the glottis (*C*). There is a bulky supraglottic mass with involvement of the pre-epiglottic and paraglottic spaces (*arrows in A and B*). At the level of the glottis (*arrows in C*), no abnormal tissue is seen; tumor is confined to the supraglottic larynx (T3) and is amenable to partial supraglottic laryngectomy.

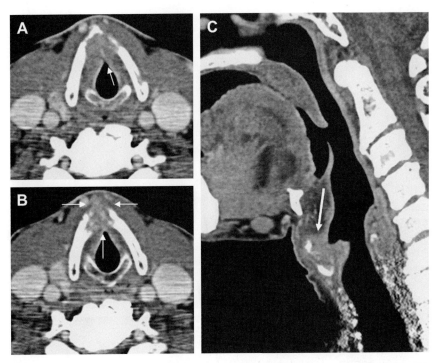

Fig. 4. (*A, B*) Axial CT images show a relatively small tumor in the anterior commissure with destruction of the thyroid cartilage and extralaryngeal extension (*arrows*). The submucosal extent of the tumor was not apparent to the surgeon. (*C*) There is also marginal extension to the caudal aspect of the pre-epiglottic space, which is best seen on sagittal CT (*arrow*).

posterior commissures, which are bounded by air inside and cartilage outside, simplifying the detection of tumor involvement. If no tissue is seen in these regions, tumor extension can reliably be excluded. When there is visible soft tissue in the region of the anterior or posterior commissure, tumor infiltration is considered, although physiologic apposition of the vocal cords and edema can give a similar appearance. Simple bulging of the vocal cord mass into these regions should not be overinterpreted as invasion (Fig. 6). Endoscopic evaluation of the mucosal extent of disease in the anterior and posterior commissures is more reliable than imaging; however, submucosal extent, particularly in the form of thyroid cartilage invasion or extension through the cricothyroid membrane, is common once the anterior commissure is involved and often escapes clinical detection (see Fig. 4). Extension of a vocal cord tumor to the anterior commissure does not change the T-staging but may affect survival and choice of treatment method, because surgical exposure of this region with endoscopic tools may be challenging and vertical laryngectomies would require a more extended approach. Involvement of the posterior commissure constitutes a contraindication for supracricoid partial laryngectomy.

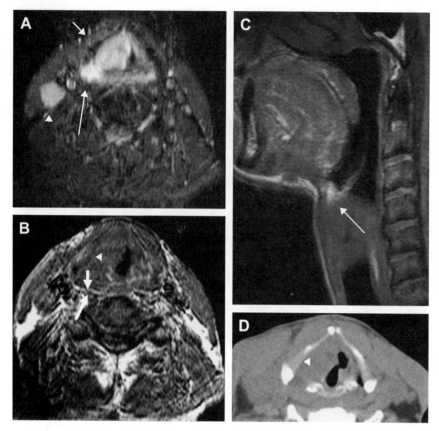

Fig. 5. Supraglottic cancer that grew anteriorly into the pre-epiglottic space is best seen on a sagittal T1-weighted image as replacement of bright fat in this region (*C, arrow*) and in the paraglottic region as demonstrated on T2-weighted axial MRI (*A, arrows*). Tumor posteriorly extends into the cricothyroid gap and bulges to the prevertebral region. (*B*) Preservation of the retropharyngeal bright fat stripe seen on an axial T1-weighted image (*arrow*) indicates lack of extension to the prevertebral space. (*D*) Tumor abuts the thyroid cartilage, which is completely ossified (*arrowhead*). (*B*) On the corresponding axial T1-weighted image, preservation of the fatty marrow signal and dark signal from the cortex is demonstrated (*arrowhead*) despite the heterogeneity created by incomplete ossification, indicating lack of cartilage involvement. (*A*) Note the metastatic node in the right neck (*arrowhead*).

Subglottic spread

Imaging plays an essential role in assessment for subglottic spread of disease, because this region is difficult to evaluate endoscopically. Imaging with CT or MRI can reliably identify subglottic extension, because the subglottis normally is lined by a thin layer of mucosa. Any additional soft tissue in this region should be treated as suspicious for neoplastic involvement. This evaluation is easier in the coronal plane but can be accomplished with similar accuracy in the axial plane (Fig. 7). The conus elasticus, a tough collagenous

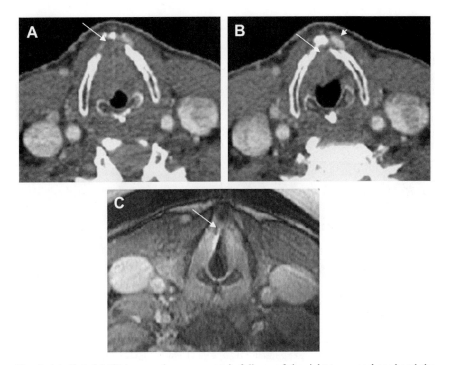

Fig. 6. (*A, B*) Axial CT images show asymmetric fullness of the right true vocal cord and the anterior commissure (*long arrows*), giving the impression that the tumor extends to the anterior commissure. (*B*) Short arrow points to the pyramidal lobe of the thyroid, mimicking extralaryngeal extension of glottic cancer. (*C*) MRI shows the anterior extent of tumor (*arrow*) without involvement of the anterior commissure. The discrepancy between the MRI and CT is likely attributable to the differences in respiratory phase during imaging. Endoscopy revealed T1 squamous cell cancer of the right true cord without anterior commissure involvement.

membrane, extends from the true vocal cord to the superior margin of the cricoid cartilage and forms the lower border of the paraglottic space. As a barrier to the spread of tumor, the conus elasticus diverts submucosal tumor extension laterally, away from the cricoid cartilage. Likewise, tumors spreading along the mucosa usually spare the paraglottic region in the subglottis because of the conus elasticus. Once tumor extends below the conus elasticus, it can infiltrate the cricoid cartilage with relative ease, making it necessary to perform a total laryngectomy. Thus, it is critical to assess tumor extent in relation to the superior ring of the cricoid cartilage (Fig. 8). Visualizing tumor within the cricoid ring is a clear indication of subglottic extension. Craniocaudal tumor extent below the free edge of the true vocal cord of 10 mm anteriorly and 5 mm posteriorly can be tolerated.

Cartilaginous invasion

Cartilaginous invasion limits the probability of adequate response to radiation [6] and increases the probability of radiation-induced necrosis.

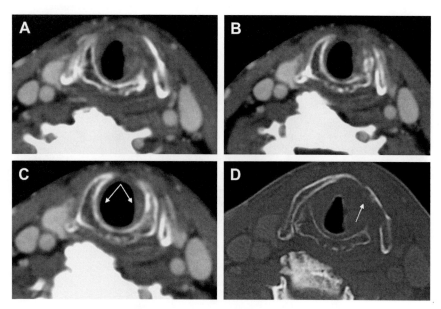

Fig. 7. Glottic cancer with subglottic extension and cartilage involvement. (*A–C*) Three axial CT images with a soft tissue window reveal subglottic extension of patient's glottic tumor. (*C*) Identification of tumor within the cricoid ring (*arrows*) indicates subglottic extension and a need for total laryngectomy. Normally, there should not be any soft tissue thicker than 1 mm in this region. (*D*) Axial CT image with a bone window through the level of the thyroid cartilage shows erosion of the inner cortex of the cartilage (*arrow*) over a large area, indicating tumor extent. Compare with the smooth surface of the right thyroid ala.

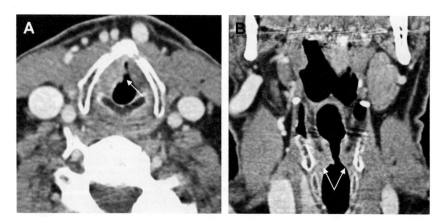

Fig. 8. Glottic cancer with subglottic extension. Axial (*A*) and coronal (*B*) CT images show a right vocal cord tumor with mucosal extent to the subglottis. Note the obscuration of right paraglottic fat density (normally present on the left side) (*arrows*), suggesting submucosal extent, but tumor does not reach the cricoid ring. A supracricoid laryngectomy was feasible.

Therefore, the presence or absence of cartilaginous invasion is an important data point for therapeutic decision making, and the presence of cartilaginous invasion often justifies extensive surgery that might not be undertaken otherwise. Because the cartilaginous structures are largely inaccessible to clinical examination, assessment of the possibility of cartilaginous invasion before treatment is the responsibility of the radiologist.

Unfortunately, the imaging characteristics of hyaline cartilage are variable. Ossification of the cartilaginous structures of the larynx increases with age but varies and may be asymmetric. Whereas ossified cartilage demonstrates high attenuation on CT at the outer and inner cortices with relatively lower attenuation, medullary space nonossified cartilage demonstrates attenuation similar to that of other soft tissue structures. On MRI, the cortical signal depends on the presence or absence of calcification, and the fatty medullary signal demonstrates T1 hyperintensity with intermediate signal on T2-weighted images. This variability can complicate imaging evaluation because of corresponding inhomogeneity of density and signal on CT and MRI, respectively, presenting a challenge to noninvasive evaluation. Further complicating matters, reactive changes within cartilage may occur without the presence of neoplastic invasion, resulting in overestimation of disease extent, particularly with MRI. Regardless, contrast enhancement is not a normal feature of cartilage on MRI or CT [7]. Either technique should be able to aid in the differentiation of inner cortical invasion (T3) from involvement of inner and outer cortices and extralaryngeal spread (T4).

As noted in the preceding discussion, MRI allows for excellent soft tissue contrast and has been viewed as superior to CT for detection of cartilaginous invasion. MRI demonstrates increased T2 signal and low to intermediate T1 signal, with abnormal enhancement in cases of replacement or infiltration of hyaline cartilage. Although these signs are quite sensitive, inflammatory and reactive peritumoral changes may have an identical appearance, limiting specificity. Some investigators suggest that inflammatory reaction may be distinguished by greater T2 signal [8]. Given the inherent sensitivity of MRI and consequent high negative predictive value, it has generally been preferred over CT at the time of initial evaluation (see Fig. 5) [7]. Recent studies, however, demonstrate that if rigorous criteria are used, more accurate information can be arrived at than previously appreciated by CT.

Becker and colleagues [9] studied the CT evaluations of 111 patients and describe CT signs with high specificity, including the presence of lysis or erosion (93% specificity) or extralaryngeal spread of neoplasm (95% specificity) (Fig. 9). Because these signs depend on relatively advanced disease, their sensitivity is understandably low. Conversely, the presence of sclerosis within a cartilaginous structure is relatively sensitive, but the specificity of this sign varies with location, being lower in the thyroid cartilage (40% specificity) than in the cricoid and arytenoid cartilages (76%–79% specificity).

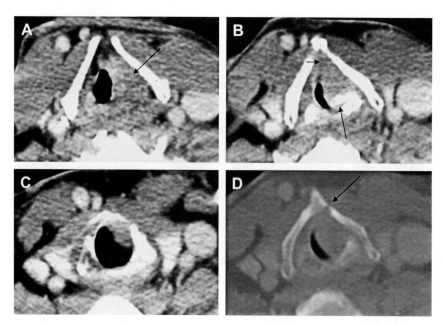

Fig. 9. Transglottic tumor with thyroid and arytenoid cartilage invasion. Axial CT images show paraglottic (*A*), glottic (*B, D*), and subglottic (*C*) tumor extension. (*A*) At the supraglottic level there is a soft tissue mass (*arrow*) replacing the paraglottic fat. (*B*) At the level of the glottis, tumor grows posteriorly to the posterior commissure. Note sclerosis of the arytenoid cartilage, indicating invasion (*long arrow*). Medial displacement of the arytenoid suggests cricoarytenoid involvement. The anterior commissure is spared (*short arrow*). (*C*) Extension of tumor to the subglottic level is obvious on imaging as normally no soft tissue thicker than 1 mm is seen in this region. (*D*) There is a focal lytic lesion in the inner surface of the thyroid cartilage (*arrow*) on bone windows that cor-responded to through-andthrough cartilage involvement on pathologic examination.

Prevertebral involvement

Involvement of the prevertebral fascia by tumor renders the tumor unre-sectable. Unfortunately, the determination of prevertebral involvement is best achieved by intraoperative observation. Radiologic detection of prever-tebral involvement is problematic. There is a small amount of fat tissue within the retropharyngeal space that can be identified on MRI and CT in most individuals. A lack of obliteration of this fat plane is a good in-dicator for lack of prevertebral involvement (see Fig. 5). Obliteration of the fat plane, conversely, does not reliably predict prevertebral tumor involve-ment unless obvious tumor bulk is present [10].

Carotid artery involvement

Unless the carotid artery is resected, extralaryngeal spread of tumor to infiltrate the carotid artery renders the tumor inoperable. Not all tumors abutting the carotid infiltrate the adventitia, however. The determination of resectable from unresectable tumors relies heavily on imaging findings.

If tumor contacts more than 270° of the circumference of the carotid, the likelihood of invasion is high and these tumors are deemed unresectable. Contact less than 180° has a low likelihood of tumor invasion. In cases with contact 180° and 270°, the radiologic distinction is not as reliable [11].

Radiologic findings and the choice of method of treatment

Preoperative assessment of resectability

Accurate assessment of tumor extension is critical in determining the method of treatment in laryngeal cancer and achieving a favorable outcome. Maintaining the quality of life is as important as achieving oncologic cure. Thus, patient preference has a significant bearing on the type of treatment chosen. In the era of an increasing variety of treatment options, including traditional surgical, minimally invasive, and nonsurgical options with voice-conserving approaches, the assessment of tumor extent with respect to certain critical structures that affect the treatment method has become even more important. Virtually all surgical and nonsurgical procedures can be modified depending on the special circumstances of each tumor.

Stage 4a tumors are generally considered resectable, whereas stage 4b tumors are not [12]. Prevertebral or mediastinal extension and invasion of the carotid artery upgrade tumors to T4b. The negative predictive value of preservation of retropharyngeal fat signal on MRI for prevertebral involvement is greater than 90%. Unfortunately, the positive predictive value of loss of retropharyngeal fat signal is approximately 60%. Thus, overall imaging diagnosis of lack of prevertebral involvement is reliable, whereas unless there is gross tumor in this region, the presence of prevertebral involvement is not [5]. As mentioned in the preceding discussion, carotid involvement can be diagnosed if the encasement of the vessel is greater than 270° and lack of invasion can be diagnosed if encasement is less than 180°. Between 180° and 270°, the accuracy of imaging is not as satisfactory [11]. Conversely, the mediastinal extent can reliably be determined by CT and MRI.

Horizontal supraglottic partial laryngectomy

A horizontal supraglottic partial laryngectomy (SPL) can be performed for many supraglottic cancers. This procedure spares the arytenoids and true vocal cords and removes the supraglottic structures, including a portion of the thyroid cartilage, with the plane of resection at the level of the laryngeal ventricles. Tumor extension below the laryngeal ventricle and substantial cartilage involvement would contraindicate this surgical procedure [13].

Supracricoid partial laryngectomy with cricohyoido(epiglotto)pexy

If there is transglottic extension of a supraglottic cancer or supraglottic extension of a glottic cancer, a supracricoid partial laryngectomy with cricohyoido(epiglotto)pexy [SCPL CH(E)P] procedure may be an option. Although the functional outcome of this procedure is not as good as that of SPL, it may be the only alternative to total laryngectomy. SCPL CH(E)P preserves at least one of the arytenoids. Contraindications to this surgical procedure include bilateral arytenoid involvement, posterior commissure disease, hyoid bone involvement, and subglottic extension beyond the upper margin of the cricoid ring. Invasion of the pre-epiglottic space is a contraindication for SCPL CH(E)P but not for supracricoid partial laryngectomy with cricohyoidopexy (SCPL CHP) [13].

Vertical hemilaryngectomy

When the tumor is confined to one side of the larynx, a vertical hemilaryngectomy may be performed. This surgical procedure removes the ipsilateral cord and up to the anterior one third of the contralateral cord as necessary. Determination of the presence and degree of extension across the anterior commissure is critical in this scenario. Contraindications include involvement greater than the anterior one third of the contralateral cord, cricoarytenoid joint involvement, and subglottic extension below the upper margin of the cricoid ring [13,14].

Lymphatic drainage of the larynx and nodal metastasis

The presence or absence of nodal metastasis at the time of diagnosis is of great importance for the prognosis of patients who have head and neck cancer. With a single lymph node involved by metastatic disease, the prognosis is said to be reduced by half. Criteria that suggest metastatic involvement of a lymph node include enlarged size, abnormal shape, necrosis, and extracapsular spread. As noted previously, nodal metastasis at the time of presentation is much more common from supraglottic carcinomas when compared with glottic and infraglottic tumors because of the rich supraglottic lymphatic network.

Lymph node staging

- N0: No regional nodal metastasis
- N1: Involvement of single ipsilateral lymph node 3 cm or less in greatest diameter
- N2a: Involvement of single ipsilateral lymph node greater than 3 cm but 6 cm or less in greatest diameter
- N2b: Involvement of multiple ipsilateral lymph nodes 6 cm or less in greatest diameter
- N2c: Involvement of multiple bilateral or contralateral lymph nodes 6 cm or less in greatest diameter
- N3: Involvement of a lymph node measuring greater than 6 cm in greatest diameter

The sensitivity of CT and MRI in detecting nodal metastasis is higher than clinical examination and lower than PET. Unfortunately, the negative predictive value of imaging, including PET, is not sufficiently high to reassure the surgeon and avoid neck dissection. Decisions regarding neck dissection in lesions staged as N0 (by imaging and examination) depend on the presumed risk for nodal metastasis and the comfort level of the surgeon and patient. The risk for nodal metastasis can be estimated on the basis of the site, depth, and extent of the primary tumor. A higher N-grading score is associated with a higher rate of treatment failure. Extranodal extension predicts a worse outcome independent of the N-grading score.

Imaging findings as prognostic indicators

It has been suggested that certain imaging findings can help to predict the prognosis of laryngeal cancer somewhat independent of the T-stage of the tumor. Virtually any imaging finding that is quantitatively related to overall tumor burden can be shown to be able to predict prognosis in a univariate analysis model [15]. More important is to identify independent risk factors among a multitude of potential risk factors. This requires multivariate analysis and is statistically more challenging. Furthermore, identification of an imaging finding is inherently a subjective phenomenon and is subject to interreader and intrareader variability. This might be a significant factor in the absence of pathologic confirmation of an imaging finding, such as is the case in tumors treated with radiotherapy. There has not been a formal investigation of the reader variability of imaging findings, with the exception of tumor volume, which can be measured with acceptable variability.

In the supraglottic cancers that are treated with definitive radiotherapy, the degree of pre-epiglottic space involvement, the degree of involvement of the paraglottic space at the level of the true cords, tumor volume, subglottic extension, and cartilage involvement can all predict the rate of local recurrence in univariate analysis. On multivariate analysis, the degree of pre-epiglottic involvement, cartilage involvement, and subglottic extension stand out as the independent predictors of local recurrence [15,16].

For glottic cancer, large tumor volume, anterior commissure involvement, ventricle involvement, and cartilage involvement are associated with higher rates of treatment failure. The only independent risk factor that is consistent among studies is cartilage involvement, which is identified by CT as inner cortex irregularity and by MRI as signal change. One study classified glottic tumors as being adjacent to and away from the thyroid cartilage inner cortex and demonstrated a worse local control rate for the lesions that contact the cartilage independent of the status of cortical irregularity [6].

Nonsquamous cell neoplasms of the larynx

Although most (>90%) neoplasms of the larynx arise from squamous mucosa, other entities are also occasionally encountered. Many malignant entities are uncommon and, with the exception of chondroid tumors, are not specifically mentioned here.

Chondrosarcoma and chondroma

The cartilaginous structures of the larynx may give rise to chondroma and chondrosarcoma, which are difficult to differentiate by imaging and even by pathologic examination. It is argued that most chondromas of the larynx are actually low-grade chondrosarcomas. It should be noted that larynx chondrosarcomas have much more favorable biologic behavior compared with extremity chondrosarcomas and that they rarely metastasize. CT is the imaging study of choice, because these lesions are distinguished from other masses on the basis of calcification of the chondroid matrix. Chondrosarcomas most commonly arise from the cricoid cartilage [17].

Metastatic disease

Metastatic disease to the structures of the larynx is quite uncommon, except possibly in late-stage disease. In the absence of prior evidence of metastatic disease, a solitary laryngeal lesion should be assumed to arise primarily from the larynx until otherwise proved.

Summary and future directions

Cross-sectional imaging of the neck is a necessary adjunct to physical examination in the evaluation of patients who have tumors of the larynx. Imaging allows for preoperative evaluation of structures that are not assessed or incompletely assessed on physical and endoscopic examination. CT and MRI remain the mainstays of preoperative assessment and provide information about the extent of disease and nodal deposits. Information provided includes the presence or absence of extent of disease to the pre-epiglottic and paraglottic spaces and the subglottis, cartilage invasion, extralaryngeal spread of disease, nodal metastasis, and tumor volume. PET-CT has a well-established role in the posttreatment setting but is not always helpful in the pretreatment stage. Further study is necessary to identify subsets of patients who have laryngeal cancer for whom PET-CT is necessary. It is hoped that tumor-specific "contrast agents" may revolutionize oncologic imaging in the future.

References

[1] Pohar S, Brown R, Newman N, et al. What does PET imaging add to conventional staging of head and neck cancer patients? Int J Radiat Oncol Biol Phys 2007;68(2):383–7.
[2] Fleming AJ Jr, Smith SP Jr, Paul CM, et al. Impact of [18F]-2-fluorodeoxyglucose-positron emission tomography/computed tomography on previously untreated head and neck cancer patients. Laryngoscope 2007;117(7):1173–9.

[3] Ljumanovic R, Langendijk JA, Hoekstra OS, et al. Distant metastases in head and neck carcinoma: identification of prognostic groups with MR imaging. Eur J Radiol 2006;60(1): 58–66.

[4] Brouwer J, Senft A, de Bree R, et al. Screening for distant metastases in patients with head and neck cancer: is there a role for (18)FDG-PET? Oral Oncol 2006;42(3):275–80.

[5] Loevner LA, Yousem DM, Montone KT, et al. Can radiologists accurately predict preepiglottic space invasion with MR imaging? AJR Am J Roentgenol 1997;169(6):1681–7.

[6] Murakami R, Furusawa M, Baba Y, et al. Dynamic helical CT of T1 and T2 glottic carcinomas: predictive value for local control with radiation therapy. AJNR Am J Neuroradiol 2000;21(7):1320–6.

[7] Becker M. Neoplastic invasion of laryngeal cartilage: radiologic diagnosis and therapeutic implications. Eur J Radiol 2000;33(3):216–29.

[8] Ljumanovic R, Langendijk JA, van Wattingen M, et al. MR imaging predictors of local control of glottic squamous cell carcinoma treated with radiation alone. Radiology 2007; 244(1):205–12.

[9] Becker M, Zbaren P, Delavelle J, et al. Neoplastic invasion of the laryngeal cartilage: reassessment of criteria for diagnosis at CT. Radiology 1997;203(2):521–32.

[10] Hsu WC, Loevner LA, Karpati R, et al. Accuracy of magnetic resonance imaging in predicting absence of fixation of head and neck cancer to the prevertebral space. Head Neck 2005;27(2):95–100.

[11] Yousem DM, Hatabu H, Hurst RW, et al. Carotid artery invasion by head and neck masses: prediction with MR imaging. Radiology 1995;195(3):715–20.

[12] Yousem DM, Gad K, Tufano RP. Resectability issues with head and neck cancer. AJNR Am J Neuroradiol 2006;27(10):2024–36.

[13] Jalisi M, Jalisi S. Advanced laryngeal carcinoma: surgical and non-surgical management options. Otolaryngol Clin North Am 2005;38(1):47–57, viii.

[14] Yeager LB, Grillone GA. Organ preservation surgery for intermediate size (T2 and T3) laryngeal cancer. Otolaryngol Clin North Am 2005;38(1):11–20, vii.

[15] Hermans R, Van den Bogaert W, Rijnders A, et al. Value of computed tomography as outcome predictor of supraglottic squamous cell carcinoma treated by definitive radiation therapy. Int J Radiat Oncol Biol Phys 1999;44(4):755–65.

[16] Ljumanovic R, Langendijk JA, Schenk B, et al. Supraglottic carcinoma treated with curative radiation therapy: identification of prognostic groups with MR imaging. Radiology 2004; 232(2):440–8.

[17] Baatenburg de Jong RJ, van Lent S, Hogendoorn PC. Chondroma and chondrosarcoma of the larynx. Curr Opin Otolaryngol Head Neck Surg 2004;12(2):98–105.

ELSEVIER
SAUNDERS

Otolaryngol Clin N Am
41 (2008) 715–740

OTOLARYNGOLOGIC
CLINICS
OF NORTH AMERICA

Radiotherapeutic Management of Laryngeal Carcinoma

Boris Hristov, MD, Gopal K. Bajaj, MD*

*Department of Radiation Oncology and Molecular Radiation Sciences,
Johns Hopkins University School of Medicine, 401 North Broadway,
Suite 1440, Baltimore, MD 21231-2410, USA*

Laryngeal cancer is the most common head and neck cancer, affecting approximately 10,000 Americans per year and accounting for almost one third of all head and neck malignancies [1]. Radiotherapy (RT) has a long and well-established history in the multidisciplinary management of laryngeal cancer, be it as a definitive local treatment for early lesions, or in combination with surgery and chemotherapy for locally advanced disease. In general, surgery and radiation are equally effective for early stage lesions, whereas more advanced stages require a multimodality approach using a combination of surgery and radiation or chemotherapy and radiation. Given the important role that the larynx plays in human speech and communication, most contemporary treatment paradigms are geared toward optimizing cure rates while preserving organ function. In addition to stage and site of disease (supraglottic versus glottic versus subglottic), treatment modality and technique also depend on a host of other factors such as age, performance status, and treatment-related side effects. A multidisciplinary approach is, therefore, essential in incorporating all of these considerations into a cohesive and effective treatment plan. This article reviews the indications for radiotherapy for cancer of the larynx and summarizes some of the important data supporting its use.

Anatomy and patterns of spread

The larynx is divided into three anatomic regions: supraglottic, glottic, and subglottic. The supraglottic larynx is composed of the supra and infrahyoid epiglottis, the aryepiglottic folds, the arytenoids, and the false vocal

* Corresponding author.

E-mail address: gopal.bajaj@inova.org (G.K. Bajaj).

0030-6665/08/$ - see front matter © 2008 Elsevier Inc. All rights reserved.
doi:10.1016/j.otc.2008.01.017

cords. The glottic larynx encompasses the true vocal cords (including anterior and posterior commissures), and the subglottic larynx extends from the lower edge of the glottis to the inferior aspect of the cricoid cartilage. The thyroid cartilage encloses the larynx anteriorly and laterally. One common pattern of spread in laryngeal carcinoma is local extension into the surrounding structures. Two important membranous barriers to local tumor spread are the quadrangular membrane, which separates the laryngeal vestibule from the hypopharynx and the conus elasticus, which is made up of fibers spanning from the cricoid inferiorly to the vocal ligament and arytenoid cartilage superiorly. In addition, the epiglottic cartilage has numerous dehiscences that facilitate tumor extension into the pre-epiglottic space, which is a fat-filled horseshoe-shaped space extending anteriorly and posterolaterally from the epiglottic cartilage. Yet another area that is vulnerable to local tumor spread is the space between the true and false vocal cords or the so-called laryngeal ventricle (or sinus of Morgagni), as this structure is not protected by the quadrangular membrane.

The most common type of cancer of the larynx is squamous cell cancer, ranging from carcinoma in situ to poorly differentiated carcinoma. Much rarer cell types include verrucous, adenoidcystic, and neuroendocrine carcinomas. Laryngeal cancer is three times more likely to arise in the glottis than the supraglottis, while subglottic cancer is extremely rare, accounting for no more than 2% of all laryngeal cancers [2]. The true vocal cords are on average 2 cm long and are thinnest anteriorly and posteriorly where they insert into the thyroid cartilage and the vocal processes of the arytenoids, respectively [3]. Most lesions arise on the free edge and upper surface of the anterior two thirds of the vocal cords, frequently extending to the anterior commissure. These tumors typically grow very slowly and remain confined to the mucosa of the true vocal cords. Larger or more infiltrative glottic tumors can invade the paraglottic and pre-epiglottic spaces, which offer little resistance to further spread through the ligaments and membranes around the thyroid cartilage or through the thyroid cartilage itself.

Local spread

In contrast to glottic lesions, supraglottic tumors have varying local extension patterns depending on which anatomic subsite they originate from. For example, suprahyoid lesions are often exophytic and can grow to a relatively large size without causing many symptoms. One important consideration is that the marked regression of these lesions after chemoradiation can compromise the anatomic integrity of the epiglottis, thus increasing the risk for aspiration. In contrast, infrahyoid lesions tend to grow anteriorly or circumferentially, whereas lesions from the aryepiglottic folds can extend in virtually all directions. Subglottic lesions spread either inferiorly to the trachea and into the neck or to the glottis superiorly. The location and degree of locoregional spread can often account for the nature and severity of symptoms at presentation, such as hoarseness, sore throat, shortness of breath, dysphagia, and throat "fullness." For example, patients with supraglottic cancers, which often grow to more advanced stages, can present with sore throat, referred ear pain (via the vagus and the auricular nerve of Arnold), or enlarged neck nodes.

Nodal metastases

In contrast to the supraglottis, the glottis has virtually no lymphatic drainage and, therefore, there is a very small risk of lymph node metastasis with T1 or small T2 lesions (Table 1). The incidence of lymphadenopathy at diagnosis is about 5% for early glottic lesions and 20% for the more extensive T3/4 tumors [3]. Additionally, according to Byers and colleagues [4], the rate of occult nodal involvement is approximately 16% in patients with T3/4, N0 disease at the time of elective nodal dissection, with the most frequently involved nodes being the upper and mid-jugular nodes. As smaller tumors grow, however, they begin to involve the supraglottic or subglottic structures, which have more extensive lymphatic networks, thus significantly increasing the risk of nodal involvement. For example, older studies have shown that 55% of patients with supraglottic cancers have clinically involved lymph nodes and that up to one half of the remaining clinically

Table 1
Staging for laryngeal carcinoma

Tis: Carcinoma in situ
T1: Supraglottis: tumor limited to one subsite of supraglottis with normal cord mobility
  Glottis: T1a, tumor limited to one vocal cord or T1b, tumor limited to both vocal cords with normal cord mobility
  Subglottis: tumor limited to subglottis
T2: Supraglottis: tumor invades more than one supraglottic subsite or glottis or region outside supraglottis without larynx fixation
  Glottis: tumor extends to supra- or subglottis and/or with impaired cord mobility
  Subglottis: tumor extends to glottis with normal or impaired cord mobility
T3: Supraglottis: tumor limited to larynx with cord fixation or invades laryngeal structures and/or erodes inner cortex of thyroid cartilage
  Glottis: tumor limited to larynx with cord fixation and/or invades paraglottic space and/or erodes inner cortex of thyroid cartilage
  Subglottis: tumor limited to larynx with cord fixation
T4: T4a, tumor invades through thyroid cartilage or invades cricoid (for subglottis) and/or tissues beyond larynx (trachea, thyroid, deep tongue muscles, esophagus)
  T4b, tumor invades prevertebral space, encases carotid artery, or invades mediastinal structures

N1: Single ipsilateral node < 3 cm	MX: distant metastasis cannot be assessed
N2: a, single ipsilateral node 3–6 cm	M0: No distant metastasis
b, multiple ipsilateral nodes < 6 cm	M1: Distant metastasis
c, bilateral or contralateral nodes < 6 cm	
N3: node(s) > 6 cm	

From Larynx. In: Greene F, Page D, Fleming I, et al, editors. AJCC Cancer Staging Handbook, 6th edition. Chicago: Springer; 2002. p. 61–5.

node-negative patients have pathologic nodal involvement on further evaluation [5,6]. Subglottic tumors have a similarly high rate of lymph node involvement, but in contrast to supraglottic cancers, which tend to preferentially involve the upper and mid-jugular nodes, they tend to spread to the lower jugular, pretracheal, and prelaryngeal (Delphian) nodes first. Based on these and other studies, it is generally accepted that patients with T3/4 glottic as well as patients with supraglottic and subglottic tumors merit comprehensive treatment of the nodal chains in addition to the primary tumor.

Distant metastases

In addition to direct extension and nodal involvement, laryngeal cancer can occasionally spread distantly, usually to the lungs and/or bones. Early studies have shown a rather low (less than 10%) overall incidence of distant metastases from laryngeal carcinoma, with supraglottic and subglottic cancers accounting for most cases. For example, Marks and colleagues [8] found that 23% of patients with pyriform sinus cancers develop metastatic disease, whereas only 1% of patients with glottic lesions fail distantly once their neck disease is controlled [7]. In addition, other investigators have reported distant metastasis rates approaching 15% in patients with primary subglottic squamous cell carcinomas [9]. A recent study from the Netherlands also examined risk factors associated with metastatic disease and concluded that lymph node involvement increases the risk for distant metastases three- to fourfold, whereas lymph node involvement with extracapsular extension increases this risk by a factor of 10 [10]. All of these distinctions are becoming increasingly important as refinements in surgical and chemoradiation approaches continue to affect better local control rates, thus necessitating new and more effective approaches of preventing and managing distant failures.

Radiotherapy for early glottic carcinoma

Both radiotherapy and voice-preserving surgery (excision, cordectomy, or hemilaryngectomy) are accepted treatment modalities for early (Tis, T1/T2 N0) glottic lesions. Even though large individual series have demonstrated comparable local control rates, there has been no direct comparison of these two treatment modalities in a prospective trial. A recent Cochrane review tried to compare the effectiveness of radiotherapy and surgery in early laryngeal cancer but concluded ultimately that there is not enough evidence to establish a clear superiority [11]. Additionally, there are no randomized data on functional outcomes after either treatment to help guide clinicians in their recommendations. In general, the choice of therapy is dictated by both the need for tumor control and the desire to preserve phonation after therapy, which in turn depend on a variety of factors, such as tumor location, volume of disease, extent of invasion, anterior commissure involvement, and nodal status. In addition, socioeconomic considerations, such as patient age, occupation, and likelihood of compliance can also inform the physician as to what treatment method may be most appropriate for a particular patient.

Carcinoma in situ (Tis)

The management of carcinoma in situ (Tis) of the glottis is controversial, with treatment practices ranging from primary radiation or surgery (vocal cord stripping, microexcision, cordectomy, or partial laryngectomy) to observation after biopsy. A few studies on the latter approach, however, have documented high rates of progression to invasive squamous cell carcinoma that is often no longer amenable to voice-preserving therapy [12]. In addition, some series have shown that, due to limited biopsy sampling, many patients with Tis actually harbor invasive disease [13]. Therefore, most physicians advocate treatment, either with minimally invasive surgery or radiation. Complete stripping of the mucosa of the cord is often curative for early dysplastic lesions (leukoplakia, erythroplakia, hyperkeratosis); however, the disadvantage with this method is that patients need careful observation and frequently require repeat procedures that may eventually scar the cords, thus obscuring new lesions and leading to hoarseness. Furthermore, many radiation oncologists believe that surgical techniques tend to be more operator-dependent than the well-established approaches and treatment paradigms with radiation, and that, unless patients are undergoing these procedures at high volume head and neck cancer centers, they should preferentially be steered toward radiation. These considerations favor RT, which has traditionally conferred excellent local control rates in the range of 85% to 100% (Table 2). In addition, surgical salvage rates after recurrence are excellent, ranging from 90% to 100%, whereas the salvage potential of radiation after surgery in early glottic lesions has not been as extensively investigated. The main disadvantages of radiotherapy are the acute side effects from treatment and the length of treatment. Also, some critics point out that most patients salvaged with surgery after recurrence require total laryngectomy and that initial treatment with surgery tends to be more cost effective [21,22].

T1 glottic lesions

Similar concerns regarding the advantages and disadvantages of surgery versus radiation stimulate the debate on the most appropriate treatment for T1 glottic lesions. In general, these lesions can also be treated very effectively with either surgery or radiation. For example, in one of the largest surgical series reported to date, the 3-year local control rates for patients with T1a and T2b lesions undergoing laser cordectomy were 94% and 91%, respectively [23]. In another large study using radiation as the treatment of choice, the 5-year local control rates were comparable at 94% for T1a and 93% for T1b tumors [19]. Because T1 lesions can be so diverse in terms of presentation, many clinicians base their treatment recommendations on ancillary

Table 2
Local control results from large recent studies of RT for early glottic cancer

Study	N	5-year local control, %
Tis		
Wang [14]	60	92
Spayne, et al [15]	67	98
Garcia-Serra, et al [16]	30	88
Cellai, et al [17]	89	84
T1		
Wang [14]	665	93
Warde, et al [18]	449	91 (T1a)
		82 (T1b)
Mendenhall, et al [19]	291	94 (T1a)
		93 (T1b)
Cellai, et al [17]	831	84
T2		
Wang [14]	237	71–77
Warde, et al [18]	230	69
Frata, et al [20]	256	73

criteria, such as lesion size, shape, location, and anterior commissure involvement. Some of these criteria, such as involvement of the anterior commissure, are thought to be poor prognostic factors that negatively impact the likelihood for local control and voice preservation after therapy [24]. The largest retrospective study on radiotherapy outcomes in T1 glottic cancer, recently published by Cellai and colleagues [17] from Italy, lends further support to these findings. A total of 831 patients with T1N0 glottic tumors were analyzed and a 5-year local control rate of 84% was reported (see Table 2). This compares favorably with local control rates from other published series, but more importantly, in this study lesion extent and anterior commissure involvement were shown to predict in a statistically significant way for local or locoregional failure on both uni- and multivariate analysis. Additionally, some investigators have reported significantly lower actuarial local control rates after radiotherapy for bulky versus small T1 lesions, lending some credence to the approach of laser excision followed by RT for more extensive T1 tumors [25]. In general, however, either RT or surgery alone is used and both are given equal consideration if the lesion is small, limited to one vocal cord (T1a), and if there is no extension to the arytenoids or the anterior commissure. However, occasionally endoscopic laser resection is recommended over RT for the well-defined superficial lesion located in the middle third of the vocal cord, particularly when it is along the cord's free edge, as RT takes much longer to administer. This recommendation is also supported by studies that have shown very similar voice quality measures in patients with mid-cord tumors undergoing limited excision as well as those receiving definitive RT for such early glottic lesions [26]. In contrast, because the surgical management of larger (especially T1b) lesions requires the removal of greater amounts of tissue with an increasing potential for poor voice quality as a result, radiation is usually the preferred initial treatment for those tumors.

Even though many clinicians take into consideration the potential for dysphonia after either mode of therapy, there are really very few good studies comparing voice quality after radiation versus laser excision. In fact, most of them are retrospective single institution series that when taken together yield conflicting impressions. On the one hand, Hirano and colleagues [27] concluded in the 1980s that hoarseness and poor approximation of the vocal cords were more frequently observed in patients treated with laser excision. Similarly, data from our institution suggested a few years later that a higher proportion of patients treated with radiation for T1 glottic carcinoma retain normal to near-normal voice quality when compared with patients treated with laser excision [28]. On the other hand, however, more recent evidence seems to contradict these findings, perhaps reflecting recent improvements in endoscopic microsurgical techniques. A recent study from Canada, for example, suggests that even though vocal cord function (as assessed by videostroboscopy) was superior in the patients who received RT, the patients who underwent endoscopic resection of their tumors actually scored higher on subjective and objective voice assessments (Voice Handicap Index questionnaire and Visipitch parameters) [22]. In addition, a recent meta-analysis of almost 300 patients with T1 glottic tumors treated either with laser excision or radiotherapy concluded that both treatment methods result in comparable levels of voice handicap [29].

Factors affecting voice quality

Other investigators have attempted to single out specific patient- or treatment-related characteristics that predict for poor voice quality after treatment. For instance, McGuirt and colleagues observed that the greater the amount of vocalis muscle resected during laser excision, the greater the decline of voice quality posttreatment [26]. As far as radiation is concerned, continued heavy tobacco exposure during RT and extensive vocal cord stripping or multiple biopsies before RT have been postulated by some to adversely affect postirradiation voice quality [30]. Others still have suggested that voice overuse during radiation may also degrade one's voice after treatment [31]. In summary, it is very challenging to discern any significant benefit of one treatment approach versus another in patients with Tis or T1 lesions of the glottis. RT continues to be one standard approach in treating these patients. Endoscopic laser excision can provide comparable local control rates and posttreatment voice quality in selected patients and has the main advantage of brevity at a potentially lower cost, being in most cases a single outpatient procedure.

T2 glottic lesions

Given that T2 lesions are by definition larger, often extending beyond the glottis or causing some impairment of vocal cord mobility, it is not surprising that these tumors are somewhat more difficult to control with either surgery or radiation. Local control rates with radiation alone range from 65% to 80%, ultimately reaching 70% to 90% after surgical salvage (see Table 2). As far as surgery is concerned, both a vertical partial laryngectomy or a partial supracricoid laryngectomy are acceptable options for bulkier and more invasive T2 lesions, especially since local control rates are excellent and preservation of vocal cord function is somewhat less of an issue once phonation has been compromised by tumor invasion. Endoscopic resection is also an option but only in selected patients with T2 glottic tumors that are small, superficial, and with normal vocal cord mobility. Nonetheless, radiation alone is still the preferred treatment approach at many institutions due to somewhat better functional outcomes. Some investigators have even shown improved rates of disease control (92% versus 72%, 5-year disease-free survival) and better voice preservation rates (89% versus 61%) for T2N0 tumors treated with concurrent chemoradiation; however, given the low incidence of distant dissemination in these patients and the potential for greater toxicity, this approach should not be routinely recommended without further validation [32].

Loco-regional control after treatment for T2 glottic cancer

The wide range in local control rates for T2 glottic cancer is, in part, due to the heterogeneity of presentations within this stage of disease. The second largest experience to date on T2 lesions treated with RT alone was recently reported by Frata and colleagues [20] who attempted to single out features associated with a poor outcome. Over 250 cases were analyzed retrospectively and a cumulative local control probability of 73% was reported at 5 years. The main determinants of inferior local control on both univariate and multivariate analysis in this study were tumor extent and impaired cord mobility. Other investigators have looked for prognostic factors in this group of patients as well and have found very similar results. For example, patients with T2 lesions treated with radiation at the Massachusetts General Hospital were found to have a slightly better local control at 5 years if they did not have impaired vocal cord mobility (77% versus 71%) [14]. In contrast, studies from the M.D. Anderson Cancer Center did not show a clear relationship between cord mobility and outcomes after RT [33,34]. Furthermore, the influence of impaired cord mobility on surgical salvage rates after radiation is far from clear and anterior commissure involvement has failed to emerge as an independent prognostic factor in this group of patients. If anything, many investigators believe nowadays that it is simply a marker of more extensive disease, which is the actual and more significant determinant of outcome [35]. What has more clearly emerged as a predictor of local control in T2 glottic cancer is the way that radiation is delivered, namely over what period of time and to what total dose. For example, investigators from Japan recently reiterated that treatment duration of 54 days or less and

RT doses 67 Gy or more correlated with significantly better 5-year local control rates (87% versus 71%, $P = .023$ and 91% versus 60%, $P = .0013$) [36].

Technical considerations

Tis, T1 lesions. As mentioned earlier, the radiation techniques for Tis and T1 lesions are pretty standard and setup is quite simple. Patients are usually treated with two 5 × 5-cm opposed lateral fields that cover the glottic larynx with a 1- to 2-cm margin. The superior border of the field is placed at the top of the thyroid cartilage and the inferior border is extended to the bottom of the cricoid. Anteriorly the field extends 1 to 2 cm past the skin surface and posteriorly it stops at the anterior edge of the cervical vertebral bodies (Fig. 1). Occasionally, the fields are turned (collimated) slightly to match the pre-vertebral line posteriorly and tilted inferiorly by 5 to 10 degrees to avoid the shoulders, especially in patients with short necks. Both Cobalt-60 and 4- to 6-megavoltage (MV) photons can provide adequate coverage of the glottis, whereas higher energy beams are generally avoided due to a greater risk of underdosing the anterior commissure. This consideration arises from a phenomenon called dose-buildup, which essentially means that higher energy beams deposit most of their energy deeper into tissues while sparing/underdosing superficial structures. Even with 6 MV there is some risk of underdosing anterior tumors, especially in very thin patients, thus necessitating the use of tissue-equivalent bolus material to allow for adequate build-up. *Bolus* is a general term used in radiation oncology that defines various ways of simulating additional tissue in the patient so that the dose can be effectively modified to cover more superficial structures (ie, skin, subcutaneous structures). Computed tomography (CT)-based planning is generally recommended to better assess dose distribution and to

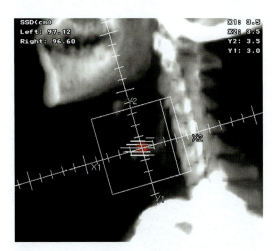

Fig. 1. Fields for a patient with a T1N0 glottic lesion. The larger field is irradiated to 60 Gy and the smaller to 66 Gy.

determine if wedges should be used. *Wedges* are beam modifiers that when placed in front of the beam allow for a varying dose distribution in tissue depending on the angle of the wedges employed. In laryngeal cancer, two 15-degree wedges are usually used to improve homogeneity and dose distribution to the mid and posterior portions of the vocal cords. Treating without wedges, on the other hand, is recommended for anterior lesions, as small hot spots in areas of disease are generally acceptable.

T2 lesions. The fields for T2 lesions are generally slightly larger to account for the greater extent of disease and the potential for supra- or subglottic involvement. They usually measure 6 × 6 cm and encompass at least one tracheal ring below the cricoid, especially if there is subglottic extension. Posteriorly, the field covers the anterior one third to one half of the cervical vertebral bodies. At our institution we also extend the superior border to 2 cm above the angle of the mandible to cover the upper jugular nodes, particularly when there is clear evidence of supraglottic extension (Fig. 2). In addition, some radiation oncologists bring in the posterior edges of their T1 and T2 fields by 1 and 1.5 cm, respectively, for the last few fractions as a way of reducing some of the dose to the pharynx. However, caution must be exercised with this technique so as not to underdose lesions that extend to the posterior glottis.

Dose of radiation. Radiation doses have traditionally ranged from 60 to 70 Gy administered in 2-Gy fractions. This approach is based on results from various studies demonstrating superior local control with fraction doses larger than 1.8 Gy (Table 3). Usually, a dose of 60 Gy is administered after surgery when there is no evidence of gross disease. For intact Tis and T1 lesions, a dose of 66 Gy has been employed, whereas T2 lesions have

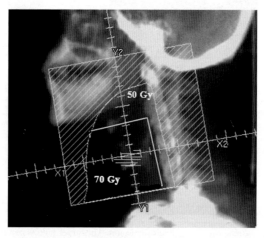

Fig. 2. Lateral fields for a patient with a T2N0 glottic lesion with supraglottic extension.

Table 3
Impact of fraction size on local control from large recent series of RT for early glottic cancer

Study	n	Stage	Radiation, Gy (dose/fraction)	5-year local control, %		P value
Schwaibold, et al [37]	56	T1	1.8	75		<.01
			2	100		
Le, et al [38]	398	T1, T2	<1.8	79 (T1)	44 (T2)	NS for T1
			≥1.8–2.24	81–92 (T1)	73–79 (T2)	.003 for T2
			>2.25	94 (T1)	100 (T2)	
Burke, et al [39]	100	T1, T2	<2	44		<.01
			≥2	92		
Garden, et al [34]	146	T2	2	59		<.001
			2.06 2.26	80		
Yamazaki, et al [40]	180	T1	2	77		.004
		T1	2.25	92		

traditionally received 70 Gy. More recently, however, several studies, including a prospective randomized study from Japan, have convincingly shown that fraction doses greater than 2 Gy are even more effective in controlling early glottic cancer than conventional fraction sizes without much added toxicity (see Table 3). For example, the Japanese study by Yamazaki and colleagues [40] demonstrated a 5-year local control rate of 92% for patients with T1 lesions receiving 2.25 Gy per fraction (total 56.25 to 63 Gy) and 77% for those receiving 2 Gy per fraction (total 60 to 66 Gy). This difference in local control was statistically significant with a P value of .004. As a result of this and other studies, some centers now irradiate with fractions of 2.25 Gy, administering total doses of 56.25 to 58.5 Gy for Tis, 63 Gy for T1N0, and 65.25 Gy for T2N0 lesions.

Nontraditional fractionation. Hyperfractionation and accelerated fractionation schemes have also been extensively investigated in both early and more advanced glottic cancer. Garden and co-investigators reported on 230 patients with T2 glottic cancer, more than a third of whom were treated with twice-daily fractionation. The 5-year local control rate was 79% for patients treated with the twice-daily regimen and 67% for those receiving once-daily treatments [34]. The largest retrospective series from the Massachusetts General Hospital also supports the use of hyperfractionation, especially in patients with T3 lesions (5-year local control 67% versus 42%, P = .03) [14]. A more recent study from Japan suggests that hyperfractionation, when compared with conventional RT dosing in T2 glottic cancer, may also improve the 5-year laryngeal preservation rate (95.3% versus 52%–60%, P < .05) [41]. In addition, hyperfractionation and accelerated fractionation schemes have also been shown to improve outcomes after radiotherapy for head and neck cancer in a few randomized trials [42–46]. For example, two of the more recent trials, Radiation Therapy Oncology (RTOG) 90-03 and the Continuous Hyperfractionated Accelerated

Radiotherapy (CHART) trials, demonstrated a benefit to altered fraction-ation for locally advanced squamous cell cancers of the head and neck but did so at the expense of added toxicity. In the RTOG trial, concomitant boost and hyperfractionated RT improved 2-year local control, disease-free survival, and overall survival when compared with standard or split-course accelerated regiments [42]. In the CHART trial, investigators compared traditional radiotherapy to a continuous regimen over 12 successive days for a total dose of 54 Gy. Even though overall disease-free survival was sim-ilar in both groups, for T3 and T4 laryngeal tumors the 3 year local control rates were significantly better with the continuous course of therapy than with conventional fractionation (70% versus 47% and 78% versus 38% respectively) [43]. RTOG 95-12, which randomized patients with T2 glottic tumors to a standard course of 70 Gy in 2 Gy per fraction or to 79.2 Gy in twice-daily 1.2-Gy fractions recently completed accrual and will hopefully add more to our knowledge of hyperfractionation in head and neck cancer.

Radiotherapy for early supraglottic carcinoma

Supraglottic carcinoma is second in incidence after glottic cancer and car-ries a somewhat poorer prognosis. The treatment options for early supra-glottic lesions (T1-2N0) include total laryngectomy, supraglottic laryngectomy, or definitive radiotherapy, with the latter two being voice-preserving and, therefore, preferred. Surgical control rates range from 80% to 90%, whereas most radiotherapy series cite local control rates between 76% and 100% depending on T stage and various other prognostic factors [2]. Traditionally, local control rates for radiation have been some-what lower than for surgery; however, direct comparisons of the two treat-ment modalities are complicated by the fact that many patients undergoing partial laryngectomy subsequently receive adjuvant RT. Also, because the leading complication of surgery is aspiration, most surgical candidates tend to be younger and healthier (eg, without evidence of COPD). Con-founding the issue even more is the higher incidence of nodal involvement, even with early stages of disease, and the resultant need for managing the neck. Comparative studies of these early lesions have noted similar rates of local control. However, they have also concluded that RT is generally associated with fewer complications and that morbidity due to chronic aspi-ration as a result of surgery can be quite high. For example, Robbins and colleagues [47] reported a 16% incidence of significant aspiration and an 8% tracheostomy rate in patients treated with a supraglottic laryngectomy. Therefore, the general recommendation is to irradiate patients with T1 and small exophytic T2 lesions, as well as patients who are medically unfit (eg, those with poor pulmonary function). All other patients with early stage disease are usually amenable to partial laryngectomy, with adjuvant RT or chemoradiation as indicated for positive/close margins, multiple positive nodes, or positive nodes with extracapsular extension.

Traditional technique

The traditional radiotherapy approach uses opposed lateral fields that extend inferiorly to the bottom of the cricoid or at least 2 cm past the lowest extent of disease. Superiorly, they encompass the larynx as well as the upper and mid jugular nodes (Fig. 3). CT-based planning is again preferred. Furthermore, to reduce the likelihood for setup errors, the patient's head and neck are immobilized during the treatment sessions with a plastiform mask (or an equivalent device), which is applied and custom-fitted at the time of simulation. Also, out of consideration for spinal cord tolerance, a shrinking field technique is used that delivers the last 13 to 15 fractions to the tumor by excluding the posterior neck and underlying cord. This is acceptable as the posterior cervical nodes are at a very low risk of involvement with T1-2N0 tumors. This smaller field still includes the upper jugular nodes and is carried to doses sufficient enough to eradicate microscopic disease. Finally, the superior edge of this field is brought down by a few centimeters to the angle of the mandible and this smaller field, which includes the lesion, and the area at highest risk for locoregional failure is then irradiated to its definitive dose (see Fig. 3).

Dose and nontraditional techniques

Patients with T1 tumors usually receive 66 to 68 Gy in 2 Gy per fraction or 63 Gy when a 2.25-Gy fractionation scheme is used. T2 lesions are given 2-Gy fractions for a total dose of 70 Gy. Nodal basins at risk are irradiated to 50 Gy using the shrinking field technique, with the off-spinal reduction occurring earlier in the treatment course at 40 to 42 Gy. Alternatively, some clinicians advocate using a hyperfractionated twice-daily regimen while others suggest an accelerated schedule with a concomitant boost.

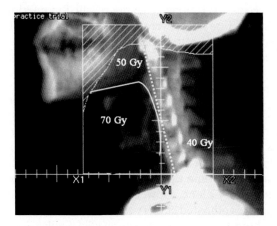

Fig. 3. Shrinking field technique for a patient with a T2N0 supraglottic tumor. Posterior low risk neck nodes are usually boosted to 50 Gy with electrons after a dose of 40 Gy is delivered with photons.

For example, investigators at the Massachusetts General Hospital analyzed 566 patients with supraglottic carcinoma, most of them with T1-3N0 disease. 244 patients received once-daily RT and 322 received twice-daily treatments. At 5 years, a statistically significant difference favoring hyperfractionation was observed in terms of both local control and disease-specific survival [14]. However, these approaches merit further investigation, as they have been shown by some to confer added toxicity [48].

In summary, even though a clear survival advantage has not been demonstrated with either larynx-preserving surgery or radiation over total laryngectomy followed by adjuvant therapy, most patients with T1 or T2 laryngeal cancer are nowadays routinely being offered larynx-preservation treatments as these are associated with significantly better functional outcomes and a better overall quality of life. Most of the current evidence supports the use of larynx-preserving techniques, either with surgery or radiation, and this approach has recently been reinforced by the American Society of Clinical Oncology (ASCO), which recommended in its 2006 guidelines that all patients with T1 or T2 laryngeal lesions be initially treated with the intent to preserve the larynx [49].

Radiotherapy for advanced glottic, supraglottic, and subglottic carcinoma

Advanced stages (T3-4 and/or N+) of laryngeal squamous cell carcinoma carry a more dismal prognosis with long-term survival rates ranging from 30% to 60% depending on the site and stage of the tumor [50]. Until 5 to 10 years ago, the traditional approach had been for patients to undergo surgery followed by RT or RT alone if they were deemed medically inoperable. These two approaches have recently been challenged by the desire to improve functional outcomes by minimizing the extent of surgery on the one hand, and because RT alone generally resulted in inferior survival rates on the other. In addition, there were many concerns about the effectiveness of RT in the postoperative setting because of tumor hypoxia and other factors fostering resistance to radiation.

Role of chemotherapy

As a result of these limitations, organ-sparing approaches with concomitant chemotherapy and radiation began to be used and studied. A major advantage of this approach was the synergistic effect of the two treatments on the tumor and the potential for early eradication of micrometastases. There are no good data concerning the effect of these strategies on survival when compared with surgery alone. However, a recently published randomized trial from Singapore compared surgery followed by RT with chemoradiation and found that both treatment strategies yielded similar 3-year disease-free survival rates in patients with stage III and IV non-nasopharyngeal and non-salivary resectable squamous cell head and neck cancers. Interestingly, those patients with laryngeal/hypopharyngeal disease subsites had a higher organ-preservation rate than the other patients (62% versus 30%) [51]. In addition, a few randomized trials have been conducted using chemotherapy and radiation as substitutes for surgery in patients with otherwise resectable laryngeal tumors. One of these, the Intergroup RTOG 91-11 trial, clearly established the superiority of chemoradiation over RT alone in terms of both local control and laryngectomy-free survival. It randomized 547 patients with potentially resectable stage III or IV laryngeal cancer to RT alone, induction chemotherapy (cisplatin/5-FU) followed by RT, or concurrent chemoradiation (cisplatin every 3 weeks). The primary end point was laryngectomy-free survival (LFS) and all patients with N2 disease underwent a scheduled neck dissection within 8 weeks of RT. Even though overall survival was identical in the three groups, at a median follow-up of almost 4 years the LFS was significantly better in the chemoradiation arm when compared with RT followed by neoadjuvant chemo or to RT alone (88% versus 75% versus 70%). In addition, local control at 2 years was also significantly better for the chemoradiation group (78% versus 61% versus 56%) and chemotherapy was shown to suppress distant metastases and improve disease-free survival [52]. In their 5-year update of these data, Forastiere and colleagues [53] showed that even with longer follow-up, LFS and locoregional control rates continued to favor concomitant therapy over the two other approaches.

An earlier randomized study, the Veterans Affairs (VA) larynx trial, also supports the use of chemotherapy and radiation as a way of improving larynx preservation and overall quality of life in patients with advanced laryngeal cancer. However, unlike the Intergroup RTOG study, patients in this study were randomized to either surgery followed by RT or to chemotherapy (cisplatin and 5-FU) followed by RT. Again, even though no differences in overall survival were observed, the larynx preservation rate was 64% at 2 years for the chemotherapy and radiation arm and the patients in this arm were more likely to report an improved quality of life as a result [54].

In addition, a few other studies have shown that when compared with patients treated with total laryngectomy, chemoradiation patients reported less impairment of speech and shoulder function as a result of treatment [55]. Largely based on these and similar series, concomitant chemoradiation is currently preferred for patients with advanced laryngeal cancer. Patients whose status precludes cisplatin-based chemotherapy during radiation should be, on the other hand, considered for cetuximab administration during RT, especially since this drug is well tolerated and since recent randomized data have shown a benefit in terms of both local control and overall survival of cetuximab with radiation in patients with advanced head and neck cancers [56].

Special consideration for T4 lesions (thyroid cartilage invasion)

When recommending therapy, however, one must remember that patients with tumor extension through the thyroid cartilage (T4) have such destruction of their laryngeal structures that they are unlikely to retain good function even after a successful combined modality approach. In addition, these patients were not included in RTOG 91-11, as only 10% of patients in that study had low-volume T4 disease (excluding patients with erosion through the entire thyroid cartilage) and all would probably be downstaged by current American Joint Committee on Cancer (AJCC) classification criteria based on minimal thyroid cartilage invasion. Therefore, such patients should be preferentially referred for surgery (ie, total laryngectomy) followed by postoperative radiation. In addition to standard indications for adjuvant radiation—such as positive/close margins, multiple nodes, or extracapsular extension of disease—subglottic extension and emergency tracheostomy before RT have also been identified as risk factors for recurrence and should prompt the clinician to consider additional therapy with radiation [57,58]. Furthermore, chemotherapy, when combined with RT in the adjuvant setting, has been shown to confer an additional benefit in two large randomized trials. For example, in the European Organization for Research and Treatment of Cancer (EORTC) 22931 trial, 334 patients with operable stage III or IV head and neck cancers and risk features including positive margins, extracapsular extension, or peri-neural invasion were randomized between RT and cisplatin versus RT alone. A 5-year overall survival advantage of 13% was noted with adjuvant chemoradiation versus RT alone (53% versus 40%) [59]. Alternatively, only a trend toward improved overall survival was shown in the similarly designed RTOG 95-01, even though it also demonstrated a better 2-year disease-free survival (54% versus 43%) and locoregional control (82% versus 72%) with concomitant chemoradiation [60]. Ultimately, however, both studies documented an increased frequency of severe toxicity with the combined treatment approach, reaffirming yet again the value of careful patient evaluation and selection.

Management of nodal disease

Another complicating factor in the treatment of advanced laryngeal cancer concerns the management of the neck. Because of the high rate of nodal involvement with T3 and T4 lesions, patients with advanced disease should undergo elective treatment of the neck, even when clinically N0. Patients with N1 involvement and with a complete clinical response may be observed after chemoradiation, whereas a scheduled neck dissection is generally recommended for patients with N2 disease or greater, regardless of response to therapy. The traditional radiotherapy approach uses opposed lateral upper fields matched with a single anterior lower field, usually at the bottom of the cricoid or at least 2 cm below the inferior extent of disease. The lateral fields should encompass the larynx and upper to mid jugular nodes whereas the anterior field covers the low neck nodes (Fig. 4). A co-isocentric setup is preferred to avoid any potential for field overlap due to divergence of the

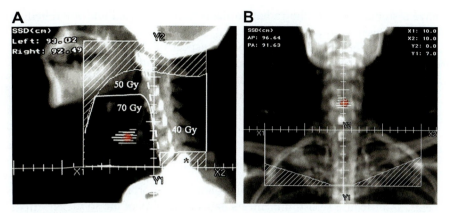

Fig. 4. Lateral shrinking fields (*A*) and anterior neck field (*B*) for a patient with T3N0 glottic cancer. In patients with advanced disease, the posterior neck is often boosted to 50 Gy with an electron field that encompasses the area posterior to the interrupted line. Also note the cord block (marked by *asterisk*) placed to prevent overlap with anterior low neck field over the spinal cord.

beams. Nonetheless, there is still some chance for overlap and a risk of over-dosing the spinal cord because of daily setup error; therefore, a small "cord block" is usually placed at the inferior and posterior aspect of the lateral fields. To further reduce this chance for setup error, the patient's head and neck are again immobilized during the treatment sessions with a plastic mask. Also out of consideration for spinal cord tolerance, a shrinking field technique is used, which delivers the last few fractions to the tumor by excluding the posterior neck. This is acceptable as a lower dose is generally needed to eradicate microscopic disease (as in clinically uninvolved lymph nodes). In advanced disease, however, this dose is insufficient and an elec-tron field is matched to the lateral photon field to administer extra dose to the posterior neck nodes at risk. This is feasible, as electrons do not have the same penetrating power in tissue as photons and cannot, therefore, deliver excess dose to the spinal cord. Usually a dose of 70 Gy in 2-Gy frac-tions is delivered to the primary tumor and involved nodes, whereas unin-volved nodes at moderate and low risk for disease receive 60 and 50 Gy respectively through the shrinking field technique outlined above.

Postoperative radiation

The traditional technique for postoperative radiation is similar to that of primary irradiation in design and setup. However, two major differences must be noted. First, the doses of radiation administered in the postopera-tive setting are usually lower if a gross total resection has been achieved. For example, patients with positive margins after surgery receive a total dose of 66 Gy in 2-Gy fractions to the tumor bed, whereas patients with negative margins are usually given 60 Gy. The second difference is that these patients have a stoma and that the radiation fields must be placed and matched in such a fashion as to adequately cover it. Occasionally, the inferior borders of the lateral fields include the superior aspect of the stoma; however, in most cases the stoma should be included in the anterior low-neck field. CT planning is particularly useful in these cases as it allows for a thorough evaluation of dose distribution and coverage. The stoma itself is usually irradiated to 50 Gy, unless there is extensive paratracheal or soft tissue extension in that region, in which case it is boosted to doses above 60 Gy.

Intensity modulated radiation therapy (IMRT)

Because the side effects from radiation are more pronounced with larger fields, and because xerostomia affects patients' quality of life so much, most patient who require extensive nodal irradiation—especially when combined with chemotherapy—are currently treated with IMRT (intensity modulated radiation therapy). This form of radiation has been greatly refined over the past few years and has, as a result, experienced an exponential growth in use. In contrast to the traditional approach, which achieves a homogeneous dose throughout the entire volume treated, this technique allows for greater conformality by delivering significantly lower doses to structures that are at low risk for disease but critical in terms of head and neck–related quality of life (eg, the parotid glands). This type of treatment requires a computer-controlled multileaf collimator (MLC) at the head of the machine, which conforms the radiation beam to various shapes (segments or subfields) throughout the course of a single treatment session. Even though there are a few different techniques to execute an IMRT plan, the ultimate goal is to create one continuous area of radiation that is made up of many smaller areas of varying intensities of radiation. In other words, this technique allows for the modulation of dose over very small distances in tissue, thus allowing for greater sparing of adjacent normal tissues (Fig. 5). The tissue-sparing effects of IMRT have been studied extensively in head and neck cancer patients and many series have demonstrated excellent efficacy in terms of tumor control with a concomitant reduction in late toxicities, particularly xerostomia. For example, Eisbruch and colleagues from the University of Michigan have shown repeatedly that saliva production is significantly affected by radiation doses over 25-30 Gy and that the use of IMRT techniques results in much less xerostomia and better long-term quality of life [61,62]. As far as laryngeal cancer is concerned, van Dieren and colleagues [63] demonstrated in a recent study that IMRT in patients with advanced supraglottic cancer can spare all salivary glands to a "considerable and probably clinically relevant degree." Additionally, preliminary data from the Memorial Sloan Kettering Cancer Center on the use of concurrent chemotherapy and IMRT in patients with advanced laryngeal cancer (mostly stage IV supraglottic tumors) recently suggested excellent outcomes with minimal toxicity. The 2-year progression-free survival and overall

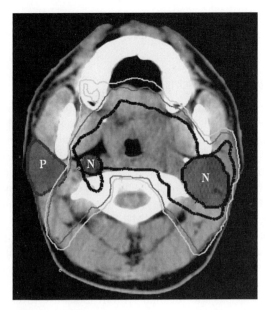

Fig. 5. An IMRT plan of a patient with advanced laryngeal cancer and extensive lymph node involvement (N). The conformal dose distribution allows for sparing of the right parotid gland (P) with the isodose lines (thick black line represents highest dose) curving around that and other uninvolved structures, such as the oral cavity anteriorly and the spinal cord posteriorly.

survival rates in this study were 90% and 69% respectively with none of the patients reporting grade 2 or greater xerostomia at the time of analysis [64].

Yet another advantage of IMRT is that one continuous area of tissue can be treated and that no field matching is required. Field matching can be problematic because of over- and underdosed areas (hot or cold spots) that can arise from daily variations in setup and that may ultimately compromise normal tissues and tumor coverage. With IMRT, most anatomic constraints, such as short necks, low-lying lesions, and stoma location, are no longer an issue and the need for field matching, with all of its inherent risks of over- and underdosing critical structures can be eliminated. With great conformality, however, comes great responsibility and as a prerequisite, IMRT requires a proper selection and a much more precise delineation of target volumes. Instead of shrinking fields to deliver varying doses of radiation, areas of high, intermediate, and low risk for disease are first delineated based on the presence of macroscopic disease and the likelihood for microscopic extension of tumor cells. Macroscopic disease usually encompasses the primary tumor and involved nodes and is irradiated to a total dose of 70 Gy in 2-Gy fractions. Intermediate- and low-risk areas are carried to 60 and 50 Gy respectively using the same fractionation schedule. Alternatively, some have successfully employed a simultaneous integrated boost approach, which delivers similar total doses to each area but does so using different fractionation schemes depending on the area at risk, thus obviating the need for a separate final boost and enabling the patient to finish treatment sooner.

Judicious use of IMRT in laryngeal cancer

Caution must be exercised, however, when using this complex modality of radiation delivery in laryngeal cancer. First, until recently, most of the studies that have investigated these alternate fractionation schemes and the effectiveness of IMRT in head and neck cancer have preferentially included patients with nasopharyngeal and oropharyngeal tumors. A major concern is that the radiobiological effectiveness of these fractionation schedules may be different for laryngeal lesions, which could adversely affect outcomes after radiation. Second, IMRT has recently been shown to lead to more regional misses and recurrences when used in early glottic lesions. A very recent editorial on this subject matter emphasizes that the primary function of IMRT is to spare the major salivary glands (specifically the parotids) and that for most patients with early carcinoma of the glottis, this is not an issue, as the regional lymph nodes are rarely involved and thus not treated [65]. IMRT should, therefore, be reserved only for patients with advanced squamous cell carcinoma of the larynx, and even in these instances it should be employed judiciously and with the understanding that further studies are needed to validate its use in this site. Finally, additional considerations, such as the higher cost of IMRT and the longer treatment sessions associated with it, must also be considered when recommending this form of RT.

Verrucous carcinoma

Verrucous carcinoma is a relatively rare variant of squamous cell carcinoma and accounts for no more than 4% of all laryngeal carcinomas [2]. These lesions are exophytic, well circumscribed, and rarely involve the lymph nodes. The use of RT to treat these lesions is controversial, as some early studies have documented that these tumors are relatively radioresistant and that they have a tendency for anaplastic transformation following RT [66]. Even though there are no firm data to support these claims, a few investigators have subsequently confirmed that the local control rate for verrucous carcinoma treated with RT is inferior to that achieved with surgical resection [67]. Based of these and other data, we recommend that early and well-lateralized tumors be surgically removed. If, however, the tumor is advanced, the patient is not a surgical candidate, or total laryngectomy is the only option, radiation can be used with the understanding that 5-year local control rates are in the order of only 50% to 60%, even for early lesions, and that close subsequent monitoring should be undertaken.

Radiation-related morbidity

The side effects from radiation are dependent upon the dose, the fraction size, the radiation volume, and the concurrent use of chemotherapy, and can, for all practical purposes, be divided into acute and late effects.

Early laryngeal lesions (Tis, T1, T2)

Because the amount of normal tissue in the treatment port for early T1 or T2 glottic carcinoma is rather small, RT for these lesions is most commonly associated with only mild and transient side effects. Acutely, patients may experience worsening hoarseness, fatigue, and sore throat, especially toward the end of radiation. These complications usually subside within 6 to 8 weeks of radiotherapy completion and can be managed conservatively during radiation with topical anesthetics, opioids, oral rinse solutions, and anti-inflammatory agents. Late effects in these patients are rare and mostly related to voice and swallowing quality due to mild fibrosis of the laryngeal structures. However, more severe complications, such as soft tissue/cartilage necrosis and laryngeal edema, webbing, or stenosis have also been reported. For example, investigators at the M.D. Anderson Cancer Center analyzed more than 100 patients with T2 glottic tumors treated with RT and reported a 4.6% actuarial incidence of these complications at 5 years [34]. It is important to note here that continued laryngeal edema for more than 3 months after therapy must be biopsied, as it could be a sign of persistent or recurrent tumor.

Advanced laryngeal cancer

In contrast to early laryngeal cancer, advanced disease requires the treatment of nodal drainage basins and, hence, of a larger total volume. In addition, most of these patients also receive concurrent chemotherapy, which sensitizes tumor cells and normal cells alike to the effects of radiation, thereby significantly increasing the risk for acute and late toxicities. For example, many studies have shown mucositis and esophagitis to be the most prevalent acute side effects, with a reported frequency between 10% and 25% [43,68]. These side effects can be quite detrimental as they often compromise patients' nutritional status during therapy, which in turn leads to a vicious cycle of worsening mucositis (from inability to heal) and further malnutrition. It is, therefore, of the utmost importance to approach these patients in a multidisciplinary fashion from the beginning and to arrange for an assessment by the nutritionist and subsequently by gastroenterology if a feeding tube is deemed necessary. In our experience, the prophylactic placement of a feeding tube has allowed many of our patients to maintain a stable weight throughout treatment and, as a result, to minimize treatment breaks during radiation.

Long-term morbidity

Swallowing dysfunction

Long-term swallowing dysfunction as a result of chemoradiation has also been described and has recently attracted greater attention. Velopharyngeal dysfunction is now thought to be exacerbated by unnecessary irradiation of the uninvolved larynx, cricopharyngeal inlet, and cervical esophagus, prompting many clinicians and investigators to use various techniques (eg, IMRT, midline blocks, and others) to minimize dose to these important structures. Even though clinical data in this area are limited, Eisbruch and colleagues [69] have recently developed IMRT planning guidelines in an attempt to limit irradiation of various structures thought to be associated with long-term swallowing dysfunction and aspiration. Furthermore, other investigators have demonstrated some benefit with therapeutic swallowing interventions and advocate various swallowing exercises during and immediately following chemoradiation to maintain and improve long-term swallowing ability [70]

Xerostomia

As far as other long-term complications are concerned, xerostomia and thyroid dysfunction are perhaps the most important and well recognized. With the use of traditional opposed lateral fields, parotid and submandibular gland sparing is minimal at best, and xerostomia rates can be as high as 80% according to some series [43]. Even though multiple agents such as pilocarpine and amifostine have been used as a means of improving salivary function and preventing xerostomia, the data on their efficacy are ambivalent at best and many of these drugs have additional side effects. Furthermore, great progress has been made over the past few years in adequately sparing the parotid glands from excess dose through the use of IMRT planning. As a result of the continued refinement and adoption of this technology, the role of currently marketed cytoprotective agents has diminished somewhat at our institution.

Hypothyroidism

Another important late complication of RT is hypothyroidism. Based on recent evidence, the incidence of hypothyroidism after radiation appears to be much higher than generally reported. For example, Mercado and colleagues [71] demonstrated an incidence of 48% at 5 years with a median time to developing the condition of 1.4 years. A more recent study reported similar results with an overall hypothyroidism incidence after radiation of 37% [72]. Hypothyroidism is a significant complication of treatment that, if left untreated, can result in significant morbidity and mortality, particularly in the elderly and those with preexisting heart conditions. Therefore, clinicians treating patients with head and neck malignancies should actively incorporate screening for hypothyroidism into their follow-up evaluations.

Finally, other complications as a result of radiation have been noted, including osteoradionecrosis of the mandible and upper airway obstruction from severe laryngeal edema. Fortunately, the incidence of these is much lower, even with traditional techniques, and will hopefully be further reduced with careful planning and the use of more sophisticated treatment tools.

Summary

Both definitive RT and larynx-preserving surgery offer high cure rates, excellent posttreatment functional results, and acceptable morbidities for patients with early laryngeal cancer. As both are equally good options for these patients, treatment decisions regarding therapy should be made in a multidisciplinary setting based on a careful evaluation of both disease- and patient-specific parameters. The now standard and preferred approach for locally advanced laryngeal cancer is combined chemoradiation, as this method offers a chance for larynx preservation and, therewith, a chance for better function and an improved quality of life. Patients who are not candidates for this treatment should undergo surgery (usually total laryngectomy) followed by RT and chemotherapy as indicated. Even though the acute and long-term side effects of radiation can be quite severe, particularly in patients with advanced disease, novel and continuously improving methods of irradiation such as IMRT can potentially ameliorate some of these toxicities while maintaining the effectiveness of radiation as a proven treatment modality in laryngeal carcinoma.

References

[1] Ries LAG, Eisner MP, Kosary CL, et al, editors. SEER Cancer Statistics Review, 1997–2002. Bethesda, (MD): NCI; 2005.
[2] Garden AS, Morrison WH, Ang K. Larynx and hypopharynx cancer. In: Gunderson L, Tepper J, editors. Clinical radiation oncology. 2nd edition. Philadelphia: Elsevier; 2006. p. 727–49.
[3] Million RR, Cassisi NJ. Larynx. In: Million RR, editor. Management of head and neck cancer: a multidisciplinary approach. 2nd edition. Philadelphia: JB Lippincott; 1994. p. 315–64.
[4] Byers RM, Wolf PF, Ballantyne AJ. Rationale for elective modified neck dissection. Head Neck Surg 1988;10:160–7.
[5] Lindberg R. Distribution of cervical lymph node metastases from squamous cell carcinoma of the upper respiratory and digestive tract. Cancer 1972;29:1446–9.
[6] Lee NK, Goepfert H, Wendt CD. Supraglottic laryngectomy for intermediate stage cancer: U.T.M.D. Anderson Cancer Center experience with combined therapy. Laryngoscope 1990; 100:831–6.
[7] Merino OR, Lindberg RL, Fletcher GH. An analysis of distant metastases from squamous cell carcinoma of the upper respiratory and digestive tracts. Cancer 1977;40:145–51.
[8] Marks JE, Kurnik B, Powers WE, et al. Carcinoma of the pyriform sinus: an analysis of treatment results and patterns of failure. Cancer 1978;41:1008–15.
[9] Spector GJ. Distant metastases from laryngeal and hypopharyngeal cancer. ORL J Otorhinolaryngol Relat Spec 2001;63:224–8.

[10] Oosterkamp S, de Jong J, Van Den Ende P, et al. Predictive value of lymph node metastases and extracapsular extension for the risk of distant metastases in laryngeal carcinoma. Laryngoscope 2006;116:2067–70.

[11] Dey P, Arnold D, Wight R, et al. Radiotherapy versus open surgery versus endolaryngeal surgery (with or without laser) for early laryngeal squamous cell cancer. Cochrane Review. The Cochrane Library, Chichester, UK: Wiley; 2004.

[12] Hintz BL, Kagan AR, Nussbaum H, et al. A watchful waiting policy for in situ carcinoma of the vocal cords. Archives of Otolaryngology 1981;107:746–51.

[13] Pene F, Fletcher GH. Results of irradiation of the in situ carcinoma of the vocal cord. Cancer 1976;37:2586–90.

[14] Wang CC. Carcinoma of the larynx. In: Wang CC, editor. Radiation therapy for head and neck neoplasms. New York: Wiley-Liss; 1997. p. 237.

[15] Spayne J, Warde P, O'Sullivan B, et al. Carcinoma-in-situ of the glottic larynx: results of treatment with radiation therapy. Int J Radiat Oncol Biol Phys 2001;49:1235–8.

[16] Garcia-Serra A, Hinerman RW, Amdur RJ, et al. Radiotherapy for carcinoma in situ of the true vocal cords. Head Neck 2002;24:390–4.

[17] Cellai E, Frata P, Magrini SM, et al. Radical radiotherapy for early glottic cancer: results in a series of 1087 patients from two Italian radiation oncology centers. I. The case of T1N0 disease. Int J Radiat Oncol Biol Phys 2006;63:1378–86.

[18] Warde P, O'Sullivan B, Bristow R, et al. T1/T2 glottic cancer managed by external beam radiotherapy: the influence of pre-treatment hemoglobin on local control. Int J Radiat Oncol Biol Phys 1998;41:347–53.

[19] Mendenhall WM, Amdur RJ, Morris CG, et al. T1-T2N0 squamous cell carcinoma of the glottic larynx treated with radiation therapy. J Clin Oncol 2001;19:4029–36.

[20] Frata P, Cellai E, Magrini SM, et al. Radical radiotherapy for early glottic cancer: results in a series of 1087 patients from two Italian radiation oncology centers. II. The case of T2N0 disease. Int J Radiat Oncol Biol Phys 2006;63:1387–94.

[21] Smitt MC, Goffinet DR. Radiotherapy for carcinoma in situ of the glottic larynx. Int J Radiat Oncol Biol Phys 1994;28:251–5.

[22] Mlynarek A, Kost K, Gesser R. Radiotherapy versus surgery for early T1-T2 glottic carcinoma. J Otolaryngol 2006;35:413–9.

[23] Gallo A, de Vincentiis M, Manciocco V, et al. CO2 laser cordectomy for early-stage glottic carcinoma: a long-term follow-up of 156 cases. Laryngoscope 2002;112:370–4.

[24] Marshak G, Brenner B, Shvero J, et al. Prognostic factors for local control of early glottic cancer: the Rabin Medical Center retrospective study on 207 patients. Int J Radiat Oncol Biol Phys 1999;43:1009–13.

[25] Reddy SP, Mohideen N, Marks JE. Effects of tumor bulk on vocal control and survival of patients with T1 glottic cancer. Radiother Oncol 1998;47:161–6.

[26] McGuirt WF, Blalock D, Koufman JA, et al. Comparative voice results after laser resection or irradiation of T1 vocal cord carcinoma. Arch Otolaryngol Head Neck Surg 1994;120: 951–5.

[27] Hirano M, Hirade Y, Kawasaki H. Vocal function following carbon dioxide surgery for glottic carcinoma. Ann Otol Rhinol Laryngol 1985;94:232–5.

[28] Epstein BE, Lee DJ, Kashima H, et al. Stage T1 glottic carcinoma: results of radiation therapy or laser excision. Radiology 1990;175:567–70.

[29] Cohen SM, Garrett CG, Dupont WD, et al. Voice-related quality of life in T1 glottic cancer: irradiation versus endoscopic excision. Ann Otol Rhinol Laryngol 2006;115:581–6.

[30] Benninger MS, Gillen J, Thieme P, et al. Factors associated with recurrence and voice quality following radiation therapy for T1 and T2 glottic carcinomas. Laryngoscope 1984;94:488–94.

[31] Stoicheff ML. Voice following radiotherapy. Laryngoscope 1975;85:608–18.

[32] Akimoto T, Nonaka T, Kitamoto Y, et al. Radiation therapy for T2N0 laryngeal cancer: a retrospective analysis for the impact of concurrent chemotherapy on local control. Int J Radiat Oncol Biol Phys 2006;64:995–1001.

[33] Howell-Burke D, Peters LJ, Goepfert H, et al. T2 glottic cancer. Arch Otolaryngol Head Neck Surg 1990;116:830–5.

[34] Garden A, Forster K, Wong P, et al. Results of radiotherapy for T2N0 glottic carcinoma: does the "2" stand for twice-daily treatment? Int J Radiat Oncol Biol Phys 2003;55:322–8.

[35] Sessions D, Ogura J, Fried M. The anterior commissure in glottic carcinoma. Laryngoscope 1975;85:1624–32.

[36] Nomiya T, Nemoto K, Wada H, et al. Advantage of accelerated fractionation regimens in definitive radiotherapy for stage II glottic carcinoma. Ann Otol Rhinol Laryngol 2006; 115(10):727–32.

[37] Schwaibold F, Scariato A, Nunno M, et al. The effect of fraction size on control of early glottic cancer. Int J Radiat Oncol Biol Phys 1988;14:451–4.

[38] Le QT, Fu KK, Kroll S, et al. Influence of fraction size, total dose, and overall time on local control of T1-T2 glottic carcinoma. Int J Radiat Oncol Biol Phys 1997;39:115–26.

[39] Burke LS, Greven KM, McGuirt WT, et al. Definitive radiotherapy for early glottic carcinoma: prognostic factors and implications for treatment. Int J Radiat Oncol Biol Phys 1997;38:37–42.

[40] Yamazaki H, Nishiyama K, Tanaka E, et al. Radiotherapy for early glottic carcinoma (T1N0M0): results of prospective randomized study of radiation fraction size and overall treatment time. Int J Radiat Oncol Biol Phys 2006;64:77–82.

[41] Tateya I, Hirano S, Kojima H, et al. Hyperfractionated radiotherapy for T2 glottic cancer for preservation of the larynx. Eur Arch Otorhinolaryngol 2006;263(2):144–8.

[42] Fu K, Pajak T, Trotti A, et al. A radiatioin therapy oncology group (RTOG) phase III randomized study to compare hyperfractionation and two variants of accelerated fractionation to standard fractionation radiotherapy for head and neck squamous cell carcinomas: first report of RTOG 9003. Int J Radiat Oncol Biol Phys 2000;48:7–16.

[43] Dische S, Saunders M, Barrett A, et al. A randomized multicenter trial of CHART versus conventional radiotherapy in head and neck cancer. Radiother Oncol 1997;44:123–36.

[44] Horiot JC, Le-Fur R, NGuyen T, et al. Hyperfractionation versus conventional fractionation in oropharyngeal carcinoma: final analysis of a randomized trial of the EORTC cooperative group of radiotherapy. Radiother Oncol 1992;25:231–41.

[45] Sanchiz F, Milla A, Torner J, et al. Single fraction per day versus two fractions per day versus radiochemotherapy in the treatment of head and neck cancer. Int J Radiat Oncol Biol Phys 1990;19:1347–50.

[46] Pinto LH, Canary PC, Araujo CM, et al. Prospective randomized trial comparing hyperfractionated versus conventional radiotherapy in stages III and IV oropharyngeal carcinoma. Int J Radiat Oncol Biol Phys 1991;21:557–62.

[47] Robbins KT, Davidson W, Peters LJ, et al. Conservation surgery for T2 and T3 carcinomas of the supraglottic larynx. Arch Otolaryngol Head Neck Surg 1988;114:421–6.

[48] Garden AS, Morrison WH, Ang KK, et al. Hyperfractionated radiation in the treatment of squamous cell carcinomas of the head and neck: a comparison of two fractionation schedules. Int J Radiat Oncol Biol Phys 1995;31:493–502.

[49] Pfister DJ, Laurie SA, Weinstein GS, et al. American Society of Clinical Oncology clinical practice guideline for the use of larynx-preservation strategies in the treatment of laryngeal cancer. J Clin Oncol 2006;24:3693–704.

[50] Larynx. In: Greene F, Page D, Fleming I, et al, editors. AJCC Cancer Staging Handbook. 6th edition. Chicago: Springer; 2002. p. 61–5.

[51] Soo KC, Tan EH, Wee J, et al. Surgery and adjuvant radiotherapy vs. concurrent chemoradiotherapy in stage III/IV nonmetastatic squamous cell head and neck cancer: a randomized comparison. Br J Cancer 2005;93(3):279–86.

[52] Forastiere AA, Goepfert H, Maor M, et al. Concurrent chemotherapy and radiotherapy for organ preservation in advanced laryngeal cancer. N Engl J Med 2003;349:2091–8.

[53] Forastiere AA, Maor M, Weber RS, et al. Long-term results of Intergroup RTOG 91-11: a phase III trial to preserve the larynx—induction cisplatin/5-FU and radiation therapy

versus concurrent cisplatin and radiation therapy versus radiation therapy. J Clin Oncol 2006;24:284s [abstract].

[54] The Department of Veterans Affairs Laryngeal Cancer Study Group. Induction chemotherapy plus radiation compared with surgery plus radiation in patients with advanced laryngeal cancer. N Engl J Med 1991;324:1685–90.

[55] LoTempio MM, Wang KH, Sadeghi A, et al. Comparison of quality of life outcomes in laryngeal cancer patients following chemoradiation vs. total laryngectomy. Otolaryngol Head Neck Surg 2005;132(6):948–53.

[56] Bonner JA, Harari PM, Giralt J, et al. Radiotherapy plus cetuximab for squamous cell carcinoma of the head and neck. N Engl J Med 2006;354:567–78.

[57] Klein R, Fletcher GH. Evaluation of the clinical usefulness of radiological findings in squamous cell carcinomas of the larynx. Am J Roentgenol 1964;92:43–54.

[58] Yuen A, Medina J, Goepfert H, et al. Management of stage T3 and T4 glottic carcinomas. Am J Surg 1984;148:467–72.

[59] Bernier J, Domenge C, Ozsahin M, et al. Postoperative irradiation with or without concomitant chemotherapy for locally advanced head and neck cancer. N Engl J Med 2004;350: 1945–52.

[60] Cooper JS, Pajak TF, Forastiere AA, et al. Postoperative concurrent radiotherapy and chemotherapy for high-risk squamous cell carcinoma of the head and neck. N Engl J Med 2004;350:1937–44.

[61] Li Y, Taylor JM, Ten Haken RK, et al. The impact of dose on parotid salivary recovery in head and neck cancer patients treated with radiation therapy. Int J Radiat Oncol Biol Phys 2007;67(3):660–9.

[62] Jabbari S, Kim HM, Feng M, et al. Matched case-control study of quality of life and xerostomia after intensity-modulated radiotherapy or standard radiotherapy for head-and-neck cancer: initial report. Int J Radiat Oncol Biol Phys 2005;63(3):725–31.

[63] van Dieren EB, Nowak PJ, Wijers OB, et al. Beam intensity modulation using tissue compensators or dynamic multileaf collimation in three-dimensional conformal radiotherapy of primary cancers of the oropharynx and larynx, including the elective neck. Int J Radiat Oncol Biol Phys 2000;47(5):1299–309.

[64] Lee NY, O'Meara W, Chan K, et al. Concurrent chemotherapy and intensity-modulated radiotherapy for locoregionally advanced laryngeal and hypopharyngeal cancers. Int J Radiat Oncol Biol Phys 2007;69:459–68.

[65] Feigenberg SJ, Lango M, Nicolaou N, et al. Intensity-modulated radiotherapy for early larynx cancer: is there a role? Int J Radiat Oncol Biol Phys 2007;68(1):2–3.

[66] Kraus FT, Perez-Mesa C. Verrucous carcinoma. Cancer 1966;19:108–15.

[67] O'Sullivan B, Warde P, Keane T, et al. Outcome following radiotherapy in verrucous carcinoma of the larynx. Int J Radiat Oncol Biol Phys 1995;32(3):611–7.

[68] Lee DJ, Cosmatos D, Marcial VA, et al. Results of an RTOG Phase III trial (RTOG 85-27) comparing radiotherapy plus etannidazole with radiotherapy alone for locally advanced head and neck carcinomas. Int J Radiat Oncol Biol Phys 1995;32:567–76.

[69] Eisbruch A, Schwartz M, Rasch C, et al. Dysphagia and aspiration after chemoradiotherapy for head-and-neck cancer: which anatomic structures are affected and can they be spared by IMRT? Int J Radiat Oncol Biol Phys 2004;60:1425–39.

[70] Rosenthal DI, Lewin JS, Eisbruch A. Prevention and treatment of dysphagia and aspiration after chemoradiation for head and neck cancer. J Clin Oncol 2006;24(17):2636–43.

[71] Mercado G, Adelstein DJ, Saxton JP, et al. Hypothyroidism: a frequent event after radiotherapy and after radiotherapy with chemotherapy for patients with head and neck carcinoma. Cancer 2001;92(11):2892–7.

[72] Ozawa H, Saitou H, Mizutari K, et al. Hypothyroidism after radiotherapy for patients with head and neck cancer. Am J Otolaryngol 2007;28(1):46–9.

OTOLARYNGOLOGIC
CLINICS
OF NORTH AMERICA

Otolaryngol Clin N Am
41 (2008) 741–755

Organ Preservation Surgery for Laryngeal Cancer

Ralph P. Tufano, MD*, Edward M. Stafford, MD

Department of Otolaryngology - Head and Neck Surgery, 6th Floor Johns Hopkins Outpatient Center, 601 N. Caroline Street, Baltimore, MD 21287, USA

The advent of combined chemotherapy and radiation protocols in the treatment of larynx cancer has given rise to the term *organ preservation*. It is easy to think of medical strategies such as chemoradiation or radiation alone as organ preserving. They do not intimately alter the anatomy of the larynx and hence, the physiologic function of the larynx theoretically should not be altered. Physicians who treat larynx cancer should also be aware of the wide array of organ preservation surgeries for larynx cancer. There has been a renaissance in the area of surgical management of laryngeal cancer. New technology and instrumentation have helped facilitate minimally invasive strategies for early laryngeal cancer. There also has been a renewed interest in open organ preservation surgeries. Any surgical procedure that maintains physiologic speech and swallowing functions without the need for a permanent tracheostoma should be considered as an organ preservation laryngeal surgery. A thorough understanding of these surgical options and their indications is essential to provide the most comprehensive care in the treatment of the laryngeal cancer patient. The goal of this presentation is to review the open organ preservation surgical procedures for laryngeal cancer and their indications for use. Before this can be done, one must understand the principles involved in organ preservation laryngeal surgery and how it relates to evaluating and confidently selecting surgical candidates.

Principles of organ preservation surgery

Organ preservation surgery for laryngeal cancer is an art. The art is in determining which patients are eligible for an organ preservation surgical

---

* Corresponding author.
E-mail address: rtufano@jhmi.edu (R.P. Tufano).

procedure. One must delicately balance the need for maximizing local control versus a good functional outcome. All patients with laryngeal cancer should be evaluated for organ preservation surgery from their initial visit. It is the head and neck surgeon's role to find a reason why the patient would not be eligible for an organ preservation surgical approach. Certain key principles must be systematically adhered to in determining patient eligibility [1].

The most important principle is that of local control. Survival from the index cancer is compromised if there is a local failure following radiation therapy or surgery to the glottis and supraglottis [2]. Early detection of the primary site recurrence may be difficult. Medical and surgical organ preservation modalities alter the topography of the larynx and make definitive evaluation of recurrent cancer difficult. Symptoms may be attributed to the treatment intervention or recurrent tumor, although, increasing pain, ear pain, and dysphagia are ominous signs. Repeat endoscopy and biopsy of the original primary cite is certainly warranted. CT, MR, and positron emission tomography (PET) imaging may also be helpful in elucidating recurrent or persistent cancer. Organ preservation surgical procedures should only be employed when resection of the tumor can be accomplished comfortably with local control rates approximating those of total laryngectomy.

The second principle of organ preservation surgery is to be able to confidently predict the extent of the tumor. A thorough head and neck evaluation is essential. A dynamic interpretation of laryngeal function must be made. This may be performed with a mirror or fiber-optic laryngoscope. Arytenoid mobility must be carefully assessed. Maneuvers such as having the patient cough lightly will elucidate arytenoid mobility or lack thereof. It is imperative to distinguish between a fixed true vocal fold secondary to paraglottic space invasion versus crioarytenoid joint involvement with tumor. Arytenoid immobility secondary to cricoarytenoid joint involvement with tumor is a contraindication to all organ preservation surgery. CT and MRI are useful to assess nodal disease and the extent of preepiglottic and extralaryngeal spread in large tumors [3]. CT, MRI, and PET have all been advocated to some degree in helping to identify cartilaginous invasion [4]. Pretreatment endoscopy is recommended in all patients, regardless of the treatment modality employed. Diligent endoscopy under anesthesia uses microscopic and endoscopic techniques to evaluate the extent of tumor spread. Subglottic extension is carefully assessed via apneic technique with a 0- and 30-degree laryngeal rigid endoscope. The tumor should be mapped out on a standardized image of the larynx.

The third principle is that the cricoarytenoid unit is the basic functional unit of the larynx. The cricoarytenoid unit consists of an arytenoid cartilage, the cricoid cartilage, the associated musculature, and the superior and recurrent laryngeal nerves for that unit. This is a foreign concept to most surgeons who perform vertical partial laryngectomy and supraglottic laryngectomy. The surgeons, along with the T system for staging laryngeal cancer, focus on the vocal fold rather than the cricoarytenoid unit. The paradigm shift from the vocal fold to the cricoarytenoid unit is essential for the head and neck surgeon to be able to use the full spectrum of organ preservation surgeries. It is the cricoarytenoid unit, not the vocal folds, that allow for physiologic speech and swallowing without the need for a permanent tracheostoma after organ preservation surgeries such as the supracricoid laryngectomy. As long as one cricoarytenoid unit can be preserved, the patient is a candidate for organ preservation laryngeal surgery.

It is not enough for the organ preservation surgeon to describe the extent of the larynx cancer via the T staging system. The eligibility of the patient for organ preservation surgery will be based on the extent of tumor, not the T stage. For example, one can have a T2 tumor of the glottis that involves the subglottis to the level of the cricoid. This would preclude the surgeon from entertaining thoughts of organ preservation surgery because of the high likelihood of cricoid resection in obtaining a margin. On the contrary, a T4 glottic lesion with inner table cartilage invasion at the anterior commissure is a candidate for supracricoid resection, which includes resection of the entire thyroid cartilage. The T3 lesion describes a fixed vocal fold. Again, this may be secondary to paraglottic space invasion or cricoarytenoid joint involvement. The former would be a candidate for organ preservation surgery (supracricoid laryngectomy) versus the latter, where the cricoid cartilage is involved with tumor. The T staging system is important for comparing outcomes with regard to treatment modalities but certainly does not dictate the treatment modality to be employed.

The fourth principle is one that may seem counterintuitive to many. The resection of normal tissue in organ preservation surgery is necessary to achieve consistent functional outcomes in terms of speech and swallowing. Extended vertical partial laryngectomy and extended supraglottic laryngectomy typically render a defect that each time may be new and novel to reconstruct. The defect and the reconstruction are defined each time by the margins that are necessary to achieve tumor removal. This may be responsible for the variable outcomes reported in the literature for these procedures with regard to speech and swallowing [5–10]. A reliable reconstruction for each surgery that is proven with regard to speech and swallowing outcome may put the surgeon at ease with regard to the choice of organ preservation surgery versus nonsurgical organ preservation alternatives.

Evaluation

As with any head and neck neoplasm, a thorough head and neck examination is essential. Particularly important in the evaluation of a patient for organ preservation surgery is the ability to accurately predict the surface and three-dimensional extent of the lesion (second principle). A dynamic evaluation of the larynx is necessary to determine whether the patient is a candidate for organ preservation surgery. Indirect mirror examination or flexible fiber-optic laryngoscopy help to examine the mobility of the true vocal folds and the arytenoid cartilages. Numerous authors have stated that evaluating true vocal fold mobility and arytenoid mobility were key points for the preparation of organ preservation surgery [11–16]. Glottic, supraglottic, and transglottic tumors that exhibit true vocal fold fixation and arytenoid fixation should be considered a major contraindication to organ preservation surgery. Arytenoid fixation implies malignant infiltration of the cricoarytenoid joint, cricoarytenoid musculature, or both. True vocal fold fixation without arytenoid fixation is not a contraindication to organ preservation surgery. Carefully evaluating the patient to vocalize a sustained /e/, to breathe gently, to cough lightly, and to vocalize at a higher pitch, help to elucidate the status of arytenoid mobility. One must also attempt to make the distinction between apparent vocal fold fixation secondary to weight impact of supraglottic tumors versus actual transglottic spread [17,18]. There is a statistically significant relationship between the presence of abnormal cord mobility and involvement at the glottic level. This scenario could provide an unwelcome surprise for the surgeon expecting to perform a supraglottic laryngectomy if not appreciated preoperatively.

Direct laryngoscopy under general anesthesia should be employed to help with the precise mapping of the extent of tumor. Systematic use of laryngoscopes allowing for complete examination of the laryngeal structures is essential. The subglottis can be inspected with rigid 0- and 30-degree endoscopes. Bimanual palpation should be used to assess the tongue base and thyrohyoid membrane to appreciate submucosal extent of disease and possible preepiglottic space involvement. Maintaining the hyoid bone as a means for impaction on to the remaining thyroid cartilage (supraglottic laryngectomy) or cricoid cartilage (supracricoid laryngectomy) is oncologically sound in supraglottic cancer unless tumor involves the tongue base, vallecula mucosa, or hyoid bone itself [19,20]. The hyoid bone is essential in the reconstruction following supracricoid laryngectomy. Palpation and manipulation of the arytenoid cartilages with endoscopic instruments help to ascertain mobility. Although careful evaluation often helps to confidently define the extent of gross disease, one may not fully be able to appreciate the submucosal extent of tumor until the intended organ preservation surgery is being attempted. It is for this reason that all patients must consent to the possibility of total laryngectomy, if intraoperatively the tumor extent precludes the use of organ preservation surgery.

If the tumor is bulky and partially obstructing the airway, debulking can be accomplished with a laser or powered instrumentation (debrider) to avoid a tracheostomy. This is particularly important in supracricoid laryngectomy where placement of the tracheotomy is important. Simultaneous second primary tumors of the head and neck should be searched for at this time. One may or may not elect to place a percutaneous endoscopic gastrostomy tube at this time if severe dysphagia is expected to last for more than 1 month.

CT and MRI are helpful in evaluating the primary lesion with regard to the status of the preepiglottic and paraglottic spaces, the subglottic extent of tumor, and cartilaginous invasion [3,4]. The studies are supplemental and should not supplant the clinical examination. CT is especially helpful to assess for nodal metastasis [3,4].

The general medical evaluation cannot be overly emphasized in selecting patients for organ preservation surgery. The ability of the patient to tolerate general anesthesia along with factors that may complicate wound healing must be evaluated. Particularly important is the patient's cardiopulmonary status. Aging and chronic obstructive pulmonary disease greatly increase the risk of postoperative atelectasis and pneumonia [21]. The risk of postoperative aspiration increases with procedures that most disturb the sphincteric function of the larynx. A chronic and inefficient cough, purulent sputum, and, most importantly, the inability to walk up two flights of stairs without shortness of breath, bode poorly for the patient's ability to tolerate an organ preservation procedure.

The patient's sex, occupational use of voice, social status, and nutritional status, as well as alcohol intake should be strongly considered. Patient motivation for speech and swallowing therapy should be assessed and the patient should be counseled by a speech pathologist familiar with organ preservation approaches preoperatively. The need for a temporary feeding tube and tracheostomy must also be emphasized. Overall, organ preservation surgery is not recommended if the general medical status of the patient suggests potential significant complications.

Following the approach outlined above will rarely result in the need for completion total laryngectomy (for oncologic or aspiration purposes) or permanent gastrostomy.

Open organ preservation surgical approaches for larynx cancer

The discussion of open organ preservation surgical approaches for larynx cancer will focus on vertical partial laryngectomy (VPL), supraglottic laryngectomy (SGL), and supracricoid laryngectomy (SCL). Indications, contraindications, and key technical principles will be emphasized. The goal of this section is to familiarize the physician with these open surgical options while understanding that this is but one part of the organ preservation paradigm that also includes radiation and chemoradiation protocols.

Vertical partial laryngectomy

The vertical partial laryngectomy (VPL) and its many derivations is probably the most familiar organ preservation surgery to all surgeons. Classically, the vertical partial laryngectomy involves a vertical transection at some point in the thyroid cartilage. The goal is to resect a portion of the thyroid cartilage along with tumor at the glottic level. An in-depth discussion of all modifications is best left for the surgical atlases. Most patients are left with some degree of permanent hoarseness, which obviously varies with the reconstructive technique employed. Chronic dysphagia is not common. Patients typically resume a normal diet within 1 month [22].

The oncological results are variable across T stage of lesions and from institution to institution. This may be secondary to the wide array of modifications for both resection and reconstruction. In general, the literature demonstrates good 5-year local control rates for T1a lesions. The local failure rate ranges from 0% to 11% [23,24]. Local control becomes more difficult when the tumor involves the anterior commissure. One reason may be that the vertical thyrotomy is often made "blindly" and the extent of tumor at the anterior commissure may not have been fully appreciated preoperatively. Kirchner's series demonstrated that the most common site of recurrence for lesions involving the anterior commissure was the subglottis [25]. Whole organ series have demonstrated the propensity for subglottic involvement with anterior commissure tumors [20]. It is often difficult to clear the subglottic level bilaterally in vertical partial laryngectomy.

The local control rates for T2 lesions have to be carefully evaluated. Although some reports suggest good local control for T2 lesions, these lesions typically are without cord mobility impairment and without significant subglottic or supraglottic extension. Local control rates have been typically worse for T2 lesions with cord mobility impairment or significant subglottic or supraglottic extension. Most series report local failure rates greater than 14% [25–27] and two series report greater than 20% [23,28]. The local control rates for VPL in the treatment of T3 lesions are widely variable with some series demonstrating a greater than 30% local failure rate [13,14,28–31]. T3 lesions are designated such because of cord fixation secondary to either paraglottic space invasion or cricoarytenoid joint involvement. Most versions of VPL do not fully address the paraglottic space and certainly do not address the cricoarytenoid joint.

In light of the above discussion, VPL can be used successfully to achieve local control for T1 lesions without anterior commissure involvement. Caution should be exercised with regard to implementing its use for anterior commissure lesions and extensive T2 lesions. The supracricoid laryngectomy provides a better oncologic option for T3 lesions without cricoarytenoid joint involvement [32].

Supraglottic laryngectomy

Supraglottic laryngectomy (SGL), like VPL, has a number of extensions that complicate assessing local control rates. We discuss the typical supraglottic laryngectomy that preserves both true vocal folds, both arytenoids, the tongue base, and the hyoid bone. The main oncologic contraindications to standard supraglottic laryngectomy are:

(1) Involvement at the glottic level (three-quarter SGL has been used)
(2) Invasion of the cricoid or thyroid cartilage

(3) Involvement of the tongue base to within 1 cm of the circumvallate papillae

(4) Involvement of deep muscles of base of tongue

Supraglottic squamous cell cancer is a different disease process than glottic squamous cell carcinoma in many ways. Supraglottic carcinoma has a higher incidence of occult nodal metastasis and frank nodal disease at presentation. Nineteen percent of surviviors experienced a second respiratory tract primary within 5 years after the diagnosis of supraglottic carcinoma [33]. These reasons alone tend to favor a surgical treatment of supraglottic cancer. Reserving radiation for the future, if possible, may be advantageous.

Local control rates for supraglottic laryngectomy range from 0% to 15% for T1 and T2 lesions of the supraglottis [7,34–38]. There is greater variability when SGL is used for T3 and T4 lesions [7,34–38]. These series did not elucidate the factors that were responsible for recurrence in these lesions. It is possible that unrecognized glottic level involvement for T3 lesions was a factor.

Key surgical resection steps to supraglottic laryngectomy include:

(1) Expose the upper half of the thyroid cartilage

(2) Release the pyriforms to the level of the ventricle and not to the midline

(3) Anterior commissure is localized at the anterior midpoint of the thyroid cartilage

(4) Perform an oblique cut 1 mm above anterior commissure toward superior cornua of the thyroid cartilage

(5) If the preepiglottic space is involved to the thyrohyoid membrane, leave straps over it and resect hyoid bone. If not, it is oncologically sound to leave the hyoid bone [19,39]

(6) If possible, perform a transvallecula pharyngotomy below the hyoid bone

(7) Grasp the free edge of the epiglottis and transect the aryepiglottic fold just anterior to the arytenoid on the noninvolved side

(8) At the ventricle, proceed anteriorly and split the thyroid cartilage along its anterior spine to visualize the extent of tumor and proceed with the cut on the involved side.

(9) Preserve the main trunks of the superior laryngeal nerves

It is possible to extend the resection to transect a portion or all of one arytenoid cartilage for tumor extending to the glottic level. This typically results in a challenging and often creative reconstruction to achieve glottic competency [35,40,41]. While these authors have had success with these complex reconstructions, the supracricoid laryngectomy with cricohyoidopexy provides a more established functional outcome with less variability with regard to glottic competency because the reconstruction is always the same.

The reconstruction for SGL typically varies among surgeons. One common closure technique is to drill numerous holes into the remaining thyroid cartilage at its superior edge. The tongue base is then sutured to thyroid cartilage making a shelf of tissue over the glottis [42]. A simpler approach is to use a closure similar to that used in reconstructing the supracricoid laryngectomy (Fig. 1) [1]. The goal of closure is to impact the tongue base with or without the hyoid bone onto the remaining thyroid cartilage. Three symmetric, submucosal, interrupted sutures (Vicryl 1 on a 65-mm needle) are looped around the remaining thyroid cartilage and inserted into no less than 1 cm of the base of tongue. This helps to bunch up the central portion of the tongue over the glottis and assists with diverting the food bolus into the pyriform sinus. The functional outcome is maximized when patients are selected appropriately for SGL and technical errors are avoided. The need for a speech and language pathologist familiar with SGL in the rehabilitation process cannot be overemphasized.

The supraglottic laryngectomy is an excellent means of controlling T1 and T2 supraglottic lesions. T3 lesions with vocal cord fixation imply paraglottic space involvement at the glottic level [18]. The supracricoid laryngectomy with cricohyoidopexy appears to be a better oncologic and functional option for resecting these lesions, as we will discuss.

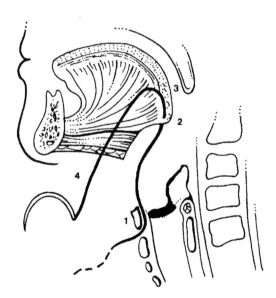

Fig. 1. Supraglottic laryngectomy reconstruction. Reconstruction in supraglottic tumor extending from false cords to the base of tongue. Resection includes the false cords, epiglottis, hyoid bone, and a portion of the base of tongue. (1) thyroid cartilage, (2) mucosa of tongue base, (3) tongue base, (4) suture exits from tongue base. (*Modified from* Weinstein GS, Laccourreye O, Brasnu D, et al. Organ preservation laryngeal surgery for laryngeal cancer. San Diego (CA): Singular Publishing Group, Inc.; 2000; with permission.)

Supracricoid laryngectomy

Although the supracricoid laryngectomy was introduced into the medical literature in 1959 by Majer and Reider [43], it has only recently begun to gain acceptance in this country. The supracricoid laryngectomy has broadened the treatment options available for treating larynx cancer by bridging the gap between the partial open procedures discussed previously and total laryngectomy. The supracricoid laryngectomy allows for excellent local control when there is strict adherence to surgical indications. It also allows for the maintenance of physiologic speech and swallowing without the need for a permanent tracheostoma.

The supracricoid laryngectomy is based on the concept that the functional anatomic unit of the larynx is the cricoarytenoid unit (arytenoids cartilage, intact cricoarytenoid joint, posterior and lateral cricoarytenoid muscles, and recurrent and superior laryngeal nerves). The preservation of one intact cricoarytenoid unit and an intact cricoid cartilage is the absolute minimum necessary to perform the operation successfully.

For selected T1b and T2 lesions, the 5-year actuarial local control estimate has been reported as high as 98.2% (61/62) [44]. Chevalier and colleagues [32] reported a 5-year actuarial local control estimate of 94.6% for 112 previously untreated patients with vocal cord motion impairment (T2 = 90) or fixation (T3 = 22).

The surgical indications for supracricoid laryngectomy include selected T1b, T2, T3, and T4 carcinomas of the larynx. The supracricoid laryngectomy also plays an important role in the surgical salvage of selected T1b and T2 radiation failures [45,46]. As we discussed earlier, surgical management is dictated by the preoperative assessment and not T staging. This concept is especially important in supracricoid laryngectomy.

Oncologic contraindications for SCL include the following:

(1) Tumors with fixation of the arytenoid cartilage secondary to cricoarytenoid joint fixation
(2) Tumors with subglottic extension to the level of the cricoid or direct invasion of the cricoid
(3) Tumors invading the posterior commissure (interarytenoid area)
(4) Tumors that extend to the outer perichondrium of the thyroid cartilage or those exhibiting extralaryngeal spread

The surgical resection is en bloc and includes the following:

(1) Both true vocal folds
(2) Both false vocal folds
(3) Both paraglottic spaces
(4) ± epiglottis
(5) Entire thyroid cartilage
(6) May include one partial or full arytenoid resection

Key surgical resection steps include the following:

(1) Blunt finger dissection along the anterior wall of trachea to facilitate reconstruction
(2) Release the pyriform sinuses from thyroid lamina as in total laryngectomy
(3) Carefully disarticulate the cricothyroid joint to avoid recurrent laryngeal nerve damage
(4) Perform a cricothyrotomy just superior to the cricoid cartilage
(5) Incise the anterior thyrohyoid membrane at level of thyroid cartilage for cricohyoidoepiglottopexy (CHEP) reconstruction (glottic tumors)
(6) Incise the thyrohyoid membrane just below the hyoid bone for cricohyoidopexy (CHP) reconstruction (transglottic tumors)
(7) Start on the less involved side and make the incision just anterior to the arytenoid cartilage, behind the ventricle and connect with the cricothyrotomy
(8) Split the thyroid cartilage at its anterior spine to give wide exposure of the tumor
(9) A partial resection of the arytenoid should be performed in patients with impaired vocal fold mobility
(10) Arytenoid resection should be performed in T3 lesions without cricoarytenoid joint involvement to clear the entire paraglottic space

The reconstruction keys:

(1) Repositioning of the pyriform sinuses and arytenoid cartilages anteriorly to facilitate postoperative swallowing
(2) Impact the hyoid bone and tongue base ± epiglottis to the cricoid cartilage using three symmetric, submucosal, sutures (1-Vicryl on 65-mm needle) (Fig. 2)
(3) Place a tracheotomy in the incision line and close the superior skin flap to the strap muscles to avoid postoperative subcutaneous emphysema
(4) If one arytenoid must be resected, preserve the posterior mucosa if oncologically possible; this will provide a buttress for the noninvolved arytenoid

The mortality rate for SCL is 1% with a postoperative morbidity rate of 11.7% [47]. A speech and language pathologist familiar with supracricoid laryngectomy is essential to maximizing functional outcome. As one would expect, the swallowing complications are slightly higher in pre- and postoperatively irradiated patients. These patients may need a prolonged feeding tube and tracheostomy compared with their untreated counterparts. Laryngeal stenosis appears to be more common in females because of a narrower cricoid cartilage [47,48]. It is also more common in previously irradiated patients and those who keep their tracheostomy tube for a prolonged period. Despite using only three sutures, the rupture of the pexy after supracricoid laryngectomy is a rare event [49].

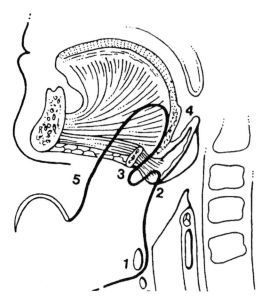

Fig. 2. Supracricoid laryngectomy with cricohyoidoepiglottopexy reconstruction. (1) cricoid cartilage, (2) base of epiglottis, (3) suture around hyoid, (4) tongue base, (5) suture exits from tongue base. (*From* Weinstein GS, Laccourreye O, Brasnu D, et al. Organ preservation laryngeal surgery for laryngeal cancer. San Diego (CA): Singular Publishing Group, Inc.; 2000; with permission.)

Conservation laryngeal surgery as salvage surgery

Total laryngectomy has traditionally been the gold standard for surgical salvage of radiation failure in laryngeal cancer. Conservation laryngeal surgery approaches are gaining wider acceptance for select patients who present with recurrence. In their 20-year review of the M.D. Anderson experience of treating radiation failures with salvage surgery, Holsinger and colleagues [50] used well-established contraindications for conservation laryngeal surgery approaches including arytenoid fixation, extensive preepiglottic space invasion, subglottic extension, and extralaryngeal spread to exclude patients who were inappropriate candidates. For those patients who were deemed good candidates, a conservation laryngeal approach instead of total laryngectomy did not cause a demonstrable change in locoregional control or disease-free survival. Other groups have reported similar results. In their review of 15 patients treated with supracricoid partial laryngectomy for surgical salvage, Spriano and colleagues [51] reported excellent long-term oncologic control. Laccourreye and colleagues [46] demonstrated a 75% long-term larynx preservation rate with 100% local control for patients treated with supracricoid laryngectomy after failed radiotherapy. With regard to open versus endolaryngeal approaches for surgical salvage, Motamed and colleagues [52] investigated this question in the literature. In their meta-analysis of all published literature on surgical salvage in laryngeal cancer, they found a preponderance of literature to support the role of conservation laryngeal surgery in the treatment of recurrent localized disease after radiotherapy. They furthermore exhibited a modest benefit of open versus endolaryngeal approaches in overall local control.

Complications in the postoperative setting are higher in those patients who have previously received radiation therapy. In radiation-naïve patients, SCPL can be performed with low morbidity and mortality. In one of the largest series published of radiation-naïve patients undergoing SCPL, Naudo and colleagues [47] demonstrated a 1% mortality and 12% local complication rate. One would expect patients who have received prior radiotherapy to fare worse. In a series of 23 patients managed with supracricoid laryngectomy for surgical salvage over a 14-year period, Makeieff and colleagues [53] found that while 17 of 23 experienced rapid functional recovery of swallowing, a significant percentage (17.4%) developed long-term swallowing impairments, with 2 patients dying from aspiration complications. Several series have demonstrated markedly increased early and late complication rates in previously radiated patients. In their series, Laccourreye and colleagues [46] had a major complication rate of 42%. Spriano and colleagues [51] described a similarly high major complication rate in previously radiated patients. A later published series by the same group demonstrated that swallowing problems postoperatively were the most common challenge in the previously radiated patient [54]. Likewise, in their meta-analysis of the literature, Marioni and others [55] found prolonged dysphagia and aspiration to be more common in radiated patients, with aspiration pneumonia and neo-laryngeal edema to be the most frequent reported postoperative complications overall. Several groups have advocated early gastrostomy tube placement in this regard [17,56]. Despite these reports, our experience of 12 patients (7 patients had one arytenoid resected) treated with SCPL for recurrence after primary radiotherapy was encouraging. There was a 92% success rate in being able to reestablish a full oral diet with removal of the feeding tube and tracheostomy tube [57].

Summary

The open organ preservation surgical procedures are an important part of the head and neck surgeon's armamentarium for treating laryngeal cancer. The principles of organ preservation surgery as they apply to laryngeal cancer must be thoroughly appreciated and strictly applied for oncologic and functional success. The selection of eligible patients for these procedures is an art and requires a keen clinical acumen. The vertical partial laryngectomy and supraglottic laryngectomy have defined clinical applications that are relatively well accepted. The supracricoid laryngectomy continues to gain acceptance as a means of treating more extensive glottic, transglottic, and early postradiotherapy lesions, while maintaining physiologic speech and swallowing without the need for a permanent tracheostoma.

The inability to include and use the open surgical organ preservation approaches in the organ preservation paradigm for larynx cancer severely limits the patient's treatment options. Total laryngectomy and medical organ preservation protocols may not be acceptable to the patient from a quality of life standpoint. Therefore, it is incumbent upon the head and neck surgeon to have a thorough understanding of all the options available for treatment in the organ preservation paradigm for laryngeal cancer. These options must be skillfully evaluated as they relate to the patient's disease process and confidently used to provide the best oncologic and functional outcome.

References

[1] Weinstein GS, Laccourreye O, Brasnu D, et al. Organ preservation surgery for laryngeal cancer. San Diego (CA): Singular Publishing Group, Inc.; 2000.
[2] Viani L, Stell DM, Dalby JE. Recurrence after radiotherapy for glottic carcinoma. Cancer 1991;67:577–84.
[3] Weinstein GS, Laccourreye O, Brasnu D, et al. The role of CT and MR in planning conservation laryngeal surgery. In: Yousem D, editor. Neuroimaging clinics of North America. Philadelphia: WB Saunders Company; 1996. p. 497–504.
[4] Castelijns JA, van de Brokel MW, Niekoop VA, et al. Imaging of the larynx. In: Yousem D, editor. Neuroimaging clinics of North America. Philadelphia: WB Saunders Company; 1996. p. 401–15.
[5] Spriano G, Antognono P, Piantaniada R, et al. Conservative management of T1-T2N0 supraglottic cancer: a retrospective study. Am J Otolaryngol 1997;18:299–305.
[6] Hirano M, Kurita S, Tateishi M, et al. Deglutition following supraglottic horizontal laryngectomy. Ann Otol Rhinol Laryngol 1987;96:7–11.
[7] Lee NK, Goepfert H, Wandt CD. Supraglottic laryngectomy for intermediate stage cancer: UT MD Anderson Cancer Center experience with combined therapy. Laryngoscope 1990; 100:831–6.
[8] Ogura JH, Sessions DG, Ciralsky RH. Glottic cancer with extension to the arytenoid. Laryngoscope 1975;85:1822–5.
[9] Flores TC, Wood BG, Levine HL, et al. Factors in successful deglutition following supraglottic laryngectomy surgery. Ann Otol Rhinol Laryngol 1982;91:579–83.
[10] Rademaker AW, Logemann JA, Pauloski BR, et al. Recovery of postoperative swallowing in patients undergoing partial laryngectomy. Head Neck 1993;15:325–34.
[11] Brasnu D, Laccourreye H, Dulmet E, et al. Mobiltiy of the vocal cord and arytenoids in squamous cell carcinoma of the larynx and hypopharynx: an anatomical and clinical comparative study. Ear Nose Throat J 1990;69:324–30.
[12] Iwai H. Limitations of conservation surgery in carcinoma involving the arytenoids. Can J Otolaryngol 1975;4:434–55.
[13] Lesinski SG, Bauer WC, Ogura JH. Hemilaryngectomy for T3 epidermoid carcinoma of the larynx. Laryngoscope 1976;86:1563–71.
[14] Biller HF, Lawson W. Partial laryngectomy for vocal cord cancer with marked limitation or fixation of the vocal cord. Laryngoscope 1986;96:61–4.
[15] Montgomery WW. Surgery of the upper respiratory system. 2nd edition. Philadelphia: Lea and Febiger; 1989.
[16] Laccourreye O, Brasnu D, Merite-Drancy A, et al. Cricohyoidopexy in selected infrahyoid epiglottic carcinomas presenting with pathologic preepiglottic space invasion. Arch Otolaryngol Head Neck Surg 1993;119:881–6.

[17] Ferlito A, Olofsson J, Rinaldo A. Barrier between the supraglottis and the glottis: myth or reality. Ann Otol Rhinol Laryngol 1997;106:716–8.

[18] Weinstein GS, Lacourreye O, Brasnu D, et al. Reconsidering a paradigm: the spread of supraglottic carcinoma to the glottis. Laryngoscope 1995;105:1129–33.

[19] Timon CI, Gullane PJ, Brown D, et al. Hyoid bone involvement by squamous cell carcinoma: clinical and pathologic features. Laryngoscope 1992;102:515–20.

[20] Kirchner JA. Two hundred laryngeal cancers: patterns of growth and spread as seen in serial section. Laryngoscope 1977;87:474–82.

[21] Evers BM, Townsend CM, Thompson JC. Organ physiology of aging. Surg Clin North Am 1994;74:23–9.

[22] Bailey BJ. Partial laryngectomy and laryngoplasty. Laryngoscope 1971;81:1742–71.

[23] Lacourreye O, Weinstein G, Brasnu DT, et al. Vertical partial laryngectomy: a critical analysis of local recurrence. Ann Otol Rhinol Laryngol 1991;100:68–71.

[24] Rothfield RE, Johnson JT, Myers EN, et al. The role of hemilaryngectomy in the management of T1 vocal cord cancer. Arch Otolaryngol Head Neck Surg 1989;115:677–80.

[25] Kirchner JA, Som ML. The anterior commissure technique of partial laryngectomy: clinical and laboratory observations. Laryngoscope 1975;85:1308–17.

[26] Liu C, Ward PH, Pleet L. Imbrication reconstruction following partial laryngectomy. Ann Otol Rhinol Laryngol 1986;95:567–71.

[27] Bailey BJ, Calcaterra TC. Vertical, subtotal laryngectomy and laryngoplasty: review of experience. Arch Otolaryngol 1971;93:232–7.

[28] Som ML. Cordal cancer with extension to the vocal process. Laryngoscope 1975;85:1298–307.

[29] Kessler DJ, Trapp TK, Calcaterra TC. The treatment of T3 glottic carcinoma with vertical partial laryngectomy. Arch Otolaryngol Head Neck Surg 1987;113:1196–9.

[30] Mendenhall WM, Million RR, Sharkey DE, et al. Stage T3 squamous cell carcinoma of the glottic larynx treated with surgery and/or radiation therapy. Int J Radiat Oncol Biol Phys 1984;10:357–63.

[31] Kirchner JA, Som ML. Clinical sign of fixed vocal cord. Laryngoscope 1971;81:1029–44.

[32] Chevalier D, Lacourreye O, Brasnu D, et al. Cricohyoidopexy for glottic carcinoma with fixation or impaired motion of the true vocal cord—5 year oncologic results. Ann Otol Rhinol Laryngol 1997;106:364–9.

[33] Wagenfeld DJ, Harwood AR, Bryce DP, et al. Second primary respiratory tract malignant neoplasms in supraglottic carcinoma. Arch Otolaryngol 1981;107:135–7.

[34] Burstein FD, Calcaterra TC. Supraglottic laryngectomy: series report and analysis of results. Laryngoscope 1985;95:833–6.

[35] Bocca B, Pinataro O, Oldini C, et al. Extended supraglottic laryngectomy: review of 84 cases. Ann Otol Rhinol Laryngol 1987;96:384–6.

[36] Alonso Regules JE, Blasiak J, de Vilaseca BA. End results of partial horizontal (functional) laryngectomy in Uruguay. Can J Otolaryngol 1975;4:397–9.

[37] Spaulding CA, Constable WC, Levine PA, et al. Partial laryngectomy and radiotherapy for supraglottic cancer: a conservative approach. Ann Otol Rhinol Laryngol 1988;98:125–9.

[38] Herranz-Gonzales J, Gavilan J, Martinez-Vidal J, et al. Supraglottic laryngectomy: functional and oncologic results. Ann Otol Rhinol Laryngol 1996;105:18–72.

[39] Bocca E. Sixteenth Daniel C. Baker, Jr, memorial lecture: surgical management of supraglottic cancer and its lymph node metastases in a conservative perspective. Ann Otol Rhinol Laryngol 1991;100:261–7.

[40] Shaw JP. Larynx and trachea in head and neck surgery. 2nd edition. London, Baltimore: Mosby-Wolfe; 1996. p. 267–353.

[41] Lawson W, Biller HF, Suen JY. Cancer of the larynx. In: Meyers EN, Suen J, editors. Cancer of the head and neck. New York: Churchill Livingstone; 1989. p. 533–91.

[42] Maves MD, Conley J, Baker DC. Laryngopharyngeal closure following supraglottic laryngectomy. Laryngoscope 1978;88:1864–7.

[43] Majer H, Reider W. Technique de laryngecomie permetant de conserver la permabilite' respiratoire la cricohyoidopexie. Ann Otolaryngol Chir Cervicofac 1959;76.

[44] Laccourreye O, Muscatello L, Laccourreye L, et al. Supracricoid laryngectomy with cricohyoidoepiglottopexy for "early" glottic carcinoma classified as T1-T2N0 invading the anterior commissure. Am J Otolaryngol 1997;18:385–90.

[45] Schwaab G, Mamelle G, Lartigau E, et al. Surgical salvage treatment of T1/T2 glottic carcinoma after failure of radiotherapy. Am J Surg 1994;168:474–5.

[46] Laccourreye O, Weinstein G, Naudo P, et al. Supracricoid partial laryngectomy after failed laryngeal radiation therapy. Laryngoscope 1996;106:495–8.

[47] Naudo P, Laccourreye O, Weinstein G, et al. Functional outcome and prognosis factors after supracricoid partial laryngectomy with cricohyoidopexy. Ann Otol Rhinol Laryngol 1997; 106:291–5.

[48] Piquet JJ, Chevalier D. Subtotal laryngectomy with cricohyoidoepiglottopexy for the treatment of extended glottic carcinomas. Am J Surg 1991;162:357–61.

[49] Laccourreye O, Laccourreye L, Brasnu D, et al. Ruptured pexis after supracricoid partial laryngectomy. Ann Otol Rhinol Laryngol 1997;106:159–64.

[50] Holsinger FC, Funk E, Roberts DB, et al. Conservation laryngeal surgery versus total laryngectomy for radiation failure in laryngeal cancer. Head Neck 2006;28:779–84.

[51] Spriano G, Pellini R, Romano G, et al. Supracricoid partial laryngectomy as salvage surgery after radiation failure. Head Neck 2002;24:759–65.

[52] Motamed M, Oaccourreye O, Bradley PJ. Salvage conservation laryngeal surgery after irradiation failure for early laryngeal cancer. Laryngoscope 2006;116:451–5.

[53] Makeieff M, Venegoni D, Mercante G, et al. Supracricoid partial laryngectomies after failure of radiation therapy. Laryngoscope 2005;115:353–7.

[54] Pellini R, Manciocco V, Spriano G. Functional outcome of supracricoid partial laryngectomy with cricohyoidopexy. Arch Otolaryngol Head Neck Surg 2006;132:1221–5.

[55] Marioni G, Marchese-Ragona R, Pastore A, et al. The role of supracricoid laryngectomy for glottic carcinoma recurrence after radiotherapy: a critical review. Acta Oto-Laryngologica 2006;126:1245–51.

[56] Clark J, Morgan G, Veness M. Salvage with supracricoid partial laryngectomy after radiation failure. ANZ J Surg 2005;75:958–62.

[57] Farrag T, Koch W, Cummings C, et al. Supracricoid laryngectomy outcomes: the Johns Hopkins Experience. Laryngoscope 2007;117(1):129–32.

ELSEVIER
SAUNDERS

Otolaryngol Clin N Am
41 (2008) 757–769

OTOLARYNGOLOGIC
CLINICS
OF NORTH AMERICA

Management of Early-Stage Laryngeal Cancer

Nishant Agrawal, MD[a], Patrick K. Ha, MD[a,b],*

[a]Department of Otolaryngology, Head and Neck Surgery, Johns Hopkins University School of Medicine, 601 North Caroline Street, JHOC 6th Floor, Baltimore, MD 21287, USA
[b]The Milton J. Dance Center for Head and Neck Cancer, Greater Baltimore Medical Center, 6569 North Charles Street, PPW Suite 200, Baltimore, MD 21204, USA

Laryngeal cancers account for almost one fourth of the approximately 45,000 head and neck malignancies diagnosed in 2007 in the United States [1], making laryngeal cancer one of the most common sites for head and neck cancer. Of these, approximately one half affect the true vocal folds [2].

Because patients who have cancers affecting their true vocal fords often present with persistent hoarseness, most are identified in the early stages: T1 or T2 [2]. In contrast, supraglottic and subglottic cancers usually do not produce early signs or symptoms; therefore, affected patients usually present with more advanced stage disease. Furthermore, unlike supraglottic and subglottic cancers, lymphatics are sparse in the glottis and metastases rarely occur in the early course of glottic cancers.

Therefore, the treatment of early glottic carcinoma is a topic of great importance and relevance. Although there is significant retrospective and uncontrolled prospective evidence that surgery or primary radiation is a good treatment option, there are no definitive, prospective, randomized controlled trials comparing the different modalities [3]. There is considerable debate on treatment of early glottic cancers with regard to local control, laryngeal preservation rate, survival, functional outcome, and salvage options for treatment failures. Regardless, given the indispensable role of the larynx in speech and communication, maintaining voice is a critical aspect in the treatment of early-stage disease. In fact, the American Society of Clinical Oncology recommends that patients who have T1 or T2 disease should

* Corresponding author. The Milton J. Dance Center for Head and Neck Cancer, Greater Baltimore Medical Center, 6569 North Charles Street, PPW Suite 200, Baltimore, MD 21204.
  E-mail address: pha1@jhmi.edu (P.K. Ha).

0030-6665/08/$ - see front matter. Published by Elsevier Inc.
doi:10.1016/j.otc.2008.01.014

initially be managed with laryngeal-preserving modalities [4]. This article reviews these management options for early glottic cancers.

Staging

Vocal fold mobility and subsite involvement are the primary determinants of glottic cancer staging. Squamous cell carcinoma of the larynx is defined by the American Joint Committee on Cancer (AJCC) [5] as follows:

Tis: Carcinoma in situ

T1a: Tumor is limited to one vocal cord with normal vocal fold mobility, including anterior or posterior commissure involvement.

T1b: Tumor involves both vocal cords with normal vocal fold mobility, including anterior or posterior commissure involvement.

T2: Tumor extends to the supraglottis or subglottis or demonstrates impaired vocal cord mobility.

T3: Tumor is limited to the larynx with vocal fold fixation, invades the paraglottic space, or demonstrates minor thyroid cartilage invasion.

T4a: Tumor invades through the thyroid cartilage or invades tissues beyond the larynx.

T4b: Tumor invades the prevertebral space, encases the carotid artery, or invades mediastinal structures.

Tis, T1, and T2 are classified under AJCC stage groupings 0, I, and II, respectively. Early-stage glottic cancers are defined as stage 0, I, or II disease, although the authors specifically address T1 and T2 disease. By definition, early-stage glottic cancers lack regional lymph node involvement or distant metastasis.

Also evident from the classification is that early-stage glottic cancers represent a diverse group of clinical disease. Early glottic cancers encompass tumors ranging from small, superficial, distinct tumors to large, diffuse, infiltrative tumors affecting one or both vocal folds. Importantly, the surgical management of these nuances is classified and standardized by the European Laryngological Society (ELS) Working Committee [6,7] as follows:

Type I: Subepithelial cordectomy—resection of the epithelium

Type II: Subligamental cordectomy—resection of the epithelium, Reinke's space, and vocal ligament

Type III: Transmuscular cordectomy—resection through the vocalis muscle

Type IV: Total cordectomy (type IV)—resection of the cord up to the anterior commissure

Type Va: Extended cordectomy—resection up to the contralateral vocal fold and the anterior commissure

Type Vb: Extended cordectomy—resection includes the arytenoids

Type Vc: Extended cordectomy—resection encompasses the subglottis

Type Vd: Extended cordectomy—resection includes the ventricle

Type VI: Cordectomy—anterior commissurectomy with bilateral anterior cordectomy

Thus, the type of resection required to eradicate the cancer may be more accurately described by the ELS types, which provide a framework in characterizing the lesions. This becomes important, particularly in publications, so that outcomes and staging can be compared more directly.

Preoperative management

Regardless of the treatment course, tissue diagnosis is mandatory to diagnose a vocal fold lesion as carcinoma. The differential diagnosis for vocal fold lesions is diverse and includes benign and malignant lesions. The methods of tissue diagnosis include an office-based brush cytologic specimen obtained through a flexible endoscope [8] or a cup biopsy with rigid endoscopy under general anesthesia. In approximately 15% to 20% of cases, a diagnostic biopsy can be diagnostic and curative [9,10]. A careful examination of the lesion should be undertaken, along with documentation of its extent. In particular, anterior commissure involvement should be noted, because this can be a difficult area to treat with surgery or radiotherapy.

The routine use of CT in early glottic cancer is probably unnecessary in T1 lesions, can be considered in T2 lesions, and should be performed in cases involving the anterior commissure. Dullerud and colleagues [11] reported that CT did not change the classification of T1 and T2 glottic tumors and concluded that imaging is required in advanced laryngeal cancers or cancers with anterior commissure involvement. In another study, CT scans resulted in changing T classification, mostly upstaging, in 21% of patients who had glottic cancers [12]. Most upstaging occurred because of subclinical involvement of the thyroid cartilage, supraglottic and subglottic extension, and soft tissue extension. Fifty-four percent of patients who had T1 disease had no abnormal findings on the scans, whereas only 20% of patients who had T2 carcinoma had negative scans. Thus, the utility of scans in T1 disease is questionable unless there are other clinical indications.

If surgery is then pursued after obtaining tissue diagnosis, further meticulous resection is required for surgical margins and depth of invasion. Alternatively, if radiation is pursued as definitive therapy, surgery is reserved for salvage therapy.

Surgery

Surgery for early glottic cancer has evolved from partial laryngectomies by means of external approaches to transoral endoscopic laser resections. Open procedures honor established principles of en bloc resection. In fact, laser excision has provided a paradigm shift in the treatment of early glottic cancer. The approach and extent of resection depend on location, size of the primary tumor, stage, and patient and physician factors. The subsequent severity of functional deficit after surgical treatment, including phonatory function and swallowing, depends on the volume of tissue resected and the resulting defect.

Transoral laser microsurgery

Steiner's [13] landmark report in 1993 exhorted the use of laser microsurgery for laryngeal carcinoma. Since then, transoral laser microsurgery has become an established time-efficient treatment option for early laryngeal cancer. Laser excision often uses a piecemeal technique compared with the standard en bloc resection. This is possible because of the magnification and lighting afforded by the use of a microscope and the specific characteristic tissue properties when dissected with the carbon dioxide (CO_2) laser.

An integral aspect of this procedure is close follow-up to detect persistent or recurrent disease on a timely basis. Based on final pathologic findings, re-excision can be accomplished and further therapy, including further laser excisions, can be considered. In a study by Jackel and colleagues [14], approximately 30% of patients who had T1 to T4 laryngeal cancer and underwent transoral laser surgery required revision laser surgery. Even though almost a third of patients required another procedure, these investigators state that the ease of revision laser surgery makes the event "unproblematic" [14]. Furthermore, most of these patients, despite pathologic reports of inadequate margins, had no residual cancer on the repeat resection specimen. If patients had residual disease on revision laser surgery, their locoregional control and laryngeal preservation rates were significantly worse but their length of survival was unaffected. Nevertheless, most patients were cleared of their disease, and only 0.7% of patients who had laryngeal cancer had persistent cancer after revision laser surgery.

Transoral laser excision is comparable to other surgical methods and radiation in terms of local control and laryngeal preservation for early glottic cancer. Several studies have reported local control rates for T1 and T2 disease in the range of 77% to 92% and 66% to 88%, respectively [15–19]. Ultimate local control after salvage therapy is approximately 97% to 98%, with a laryngeal preservation rate of 90% to 99%. The 5-year disease-specific survival rate is reported to be 90% to 98%.

Laser resection provides more therapeutic options for management of persistent or recurrent disease. Patients can be salvaged with revision laser surgery, radiation therapy, conservation laryngeal surgery, or total laryngectomy. After laser resection for early glottic lesions, tracheostomy is almost always unnecessary and diet is expeditiously advanced. There is minimal pain involved with the procedure. Additional advantages of laser surgery are short treatment time and short hospital stays [9].

Although the laser offers many advantages, safe use of the CO_2 laser mandates special awareness, training, and skill of the surgeon and operating room team. Airway fire is a potential serious complication during laryngeal laser surgery that must be avoided at all costs. Other potential complications include infection, granulomas, emphysema, cutaneous fistula, bleeding, dyspnea or shortness of breath requiring temporary or permanent tracheotomy, and dysphagia or aspiration pneumonia. The incidence of these complications is relatively rare, occurring in only approximately 4% of patients [20].

Open surgical procedures

Open surgical procedures for early glottic cancers can be regarded as organ preservation procedures because they aim to preserve speech and swallowing without a permanent stoma. Historically, open procedures required a tracheotomy. These procedures have been refined, and meticulous surgery usually obviates the need for a permanent tracheotomy. Nevertheless, patients may require a temporary tracheostomy after open partial surgery. Swallowing can be variably affected for some period, leading to wavering degrees of aspiration. Hence, patients require adequate pulmonary reserve for conservational laryngeal surgical procedures.

Several open surgical laryngeal procedures are available for the treatment of early glottic cancers [21]. Laryngofissure with cordectomy entails resection of a vocal fold through a thyrotomy. This procedure is indicated for midthird mobile vocal fold lesions. The vertical partial hemilaryngectomy, which includes removal of half of the larynx, can be successfully used for lesions without anterior commissure involvement. Other select T1 and T2 lesions, including cancers involving the anterior commissure, are treated with frontolateral hemilaryngectomy or supracricoid laryngectomy. Frontolateral partial laryngectomy removes a vocal fold, anterior commissure, anterior third of the contralateral vocal fold, and the overlying medial thyroid cartilage. Supracricoid laryngectomy preserves at least one cricoarytenoid unit and cricoid cartilage. Lesions involving the anterior commissure may involve anterior commissure procedures that remove the anterior portions of both vocal folds and the overlying cartilage.

For open surgical procedures in general, the local control rates range from 86% to 98% [16,21–25]. The ultimate local control rates vary from 99% to 100% after salvage therapy, with a laryngeal preservation rate of 88% to 100%. A 5-year disease-specific survival rate of 92% to 97% is reported for T1 and T2 lesions.

The complications after open surgical procedures depend on the procedure performed. They include formation of adhesions, granulation tissue, or stenosis; infection; cutaneous fistula; bleeding; aspiration pneumonia; gastrostomy tube dependence; tracheotomy dependence; and death.

Radiation therapy

Radiotherapy has become one of the most frequently used modalities in the United States because it offers the benefits of no surgery and has good local control and survival rates. The energies most appropriate for radiotherapy are Cobalt 60 or 4- to 6-MV photons. The typical field for radiotherapy for early glottic cancers covers the area between the superior aspect of the thyroid notch, the inferior border of the cricoid cartilage, 1 cm deep to the skin, and the prevertebral fascia [26].

Overall, for T1 and T2 lesions, the local control rates are between 82% and 87%. The 5-year disease-specific survival rate has been reported as 96% [27]. More specifically, the local control rate with radiation therapy for T1 disease is generally accepted to be approximately 90%, although there is considerable variability. Data from some of the larger studies suggest that the range is from 82% to 94% [27–33]. Most failures are surgically salvaged with ultimate local control and laryngeal preservation rates of 90% to 96% and laryngeal preservation rates of 83% to 95%, respectively. The 5-year disease-specific survival rate is 95% to 98%. Local control rates for T2 disease are in the range of 61% to 80% [27–29,31–35]. Ultimate local control after surgical salvage ranges from 80% to 91%, with a laryngeal preservation rate ranging from 60% to 82%. The 5-year cause-specific survival rate is 86% to 95%.

There is a direct correlation between the total dose and the control rate, with doses less than 65 Gy resulting in lower local control [16,25,29,30,36]. The daily fraction size also seems to be important, with 5-year local control rates of 84% to 100%, 77%, and 44% when treated with 2.25 Gy or greater, 2 Gy, and less than 1.8 Gy, respectively [29,32,37]. A prospective randomized study in Japan comparing 2.25 Gy with 2 Gy showed improved local control with the higher fraction size [38]. Logically, the duration of therapy is also important, with a treatment time of greater than 40 days associated with a local control rate of 79% to 84% versus a control rate of 95% to 100% for therapy lasting less than 40 days [29,39].

In some studies, poor prognostic factors for radiation therapy include bulky tumors [31,40], anterior commissure involvement [28,29], vocal fold motion impairment [34,41], and a larger number of subsites involved [29,31,34].

Surgical salvage after radiation treatment for persistent or recurrent cancer is a viable option. Steiner and colleagues [42] described successfully using transoral laser microsurgery to salvage radiation failures. Seventy-one percent of patients with early-stage recurrence were cured after laser surgery, with a 5-year disease-specific survival rate of 86%. Salvage surgery can also include conservational laryngeal surgery in certain cases or total laryngectomy [34,43–47]. The rate of complications, including pharyngocutaneous fistula, after surgical salvage for radiation failures is related to the dose of radiation therapy [48] and, overall, is considered to be higher.

Adverse events associated with radiation to the larynx result from early edema and mucositis and late fibrosis, xerostomia, and stenosis. Hoarseness is a common occurrence acutely and improves in most patients. Swallowing function may be altered from the fibrosis but usually also improves. Severe complications occur at a frequency between 1% and 2%, requiring a tracheotomy or total laryngectomy [27,29].

Carcinoma in situ

The treatment options for carcinoma in situ include vocal cord stripping, laser excision, and radiotherapy. Traditionally, surgical treatments are the first choice with radiation reserved for persistent recurrent disease or for widespread disease. Nevertheless, a recent meta-analysis suggests an improved local control rate with radiotherapy (94%) compared with CO_2 laser excision (81%) and vocal cord stripping (77%) [49]. These data can often be difficult to interpret, however, because of the variability between studies in pathologic staging, patient population, and extent of surgical procedure.

Anterior commissure

Approximately 20% of all glottic tumors involve the anterior commissure [50]. Despite the suggestions that anterior commissure involvement portends a worse prognosis, it is not included in the staging system. The significance of anterior commissure involvement remains controversial, however, with evidence on both sides of the argument. Some reports identify anterior commissure involvement with adverse local control, organ preservation, and survival [28–30,51], whereas other reports failed to find a significant correlation [52,53]. The anatomic affect of the anterior commissure on tumor extension is also controversial.

Steiner and colleagues [54] reported that laser surgery is effective despite anterior commissure involvement, although not all the data achieved statistical significance. Conversely, Eckel [55] showed that the anterior commissure was the most frequent site of local recurrence and discouraged the use of laser surgery. This finding may be related to the degree of exposure possible, because there can be difficulty in obtaining a clear view of the anterior commissure in some patients.

Open partial laryngectomy procedures offer good local control of tumors involving the anterior commissure at a cost of poorer voice. Laccourreye and colleagues [24] concluded that supracricoid laryngectomy with crico-hyoidoepiglottopexy for early glottic cancer with anterior commissure involvement resulted in higher local control rates and laryngeal preservation rates when compared with historical data for vertical partial laryngectomy or radiation therapy. The 3- and 5-year actuarial local control estimates were 98.2%, with one patient successfully salvaged with radiation therapy, resulting in a 100% laryngeal preservation rate.

There is mixed evidence of local control after radiation therapy for early glottic cancer with anterior commissure involvement. Mendenhall and colleagues [27] reported that there was no difference in local control at 5 years in patients with and without anterior commissure involvement. Other studies show a range of 82% to 90% 5-year local control rates in patients without anterior commissure involvement compared with a 5-year local control range of 56% to 80% in patients with anterior commissure involvement [28,29,56,57].

Given that involvement of the anterior commissure may adversely be associated with outcome, the degree of anterior commissure involvement should be defined and considered when debating treatment. Open surgical procedures may provide the best oncologic clearance.

Voice quality

Posttreatment voice quality after surgery or radiation remains controversial, and a wide range of results can be found in the literature. There are no randomized trials that have compared quality of life and voice quality in patients treated with radiation, open surgery, or laser excision. Several studies using perceptual voice measures, acoustic voice parameters, speech aerodynamic studies, or patient-based outcomes assessments have provided varying, sometimes contradictory, results. The issue is not likely to be resolved until a randomized prospective study is conducted. Until then, debates are likely to ensue.

In general, voice quality is generally believed to better after radiotherapy and worse after open laryngeal procedures. The major area of controversy is comparing voice quality after radiotherapy and laser surgery. Recently, Ledda and colleagues [58] analyzed vocal outcomes by videolaryngostroboscopy, objective, and perceptive measures. They demonstrated that patients who underwent ELS type I and II cordectomies had no statistically significant differences in the vocal parameters derived from electroacoustic analysis compared with euphonic controls. There was a statistical difference in the more extensive cordectomies, however. Casiano and colleagues [59] performed postoperative videostrobolaryngoscopy after laser surgery and found that all patients had absent or moderately reduced amplitude and mucosal wave patterns and incomplete glottic closure proportional to the volume of tissue resected, resulting in a breathy voice. Although Casiano and colleagues [59] analyzed patients who had laser surgery with or without radiation, Hirano and colleagues [60] compared patients who had laser surgery separately from patients who had radiotherapy. Their results showed that a slight degree of hoarseness, incomplete glottal closure, and reduction or absence of vibration were more frequently observed in patients after laser surgery but that there was no difference in several acoustic voice parameters and speech aerodynamic studies. Hirano and colleagues [60] concluded that regarding functional conversational speech, there was minimal difference in vocal function in the two groups. Likewise, McGuirt and colleagues [61] found no statistically significant difference between the voice quality in patients treated with laser surgery and radiation therapy. Finally, a recent meta-analysis performed in 2006 demonstrated that radiation therapy and laser excision provided similar levels of voice handicap index scores for patients who had T1a laryngeal carcinoma [62].

In summary, regardless of the treatment option, there is likely to be some alteration in the ultimate quality of voice. As such, voice therapy should be considered during or after treatment [63], especially for patients who rely heavily on their voice for career or social interactions. Hocevar-Boltezar and colleagues [64] reported some irregularities of the vocal folds after radiation therapy and poorer voice quality compared with a normal matched control group and suggested voice therapy. Finally, patients should strongly be urged to discontinue tobacco use.

Cost

The costs of the procedures are also difficult to quantify. Foote and colleagues [65] reported that the cost of radiation therapy is comparable to that of laser surgery and less than that of open surgical procedures. A European study confirmed that radiation therapy and laser surgery have almost the same average cost for the treatment for T1 squamous cell carcinoma of the larynx, whereas open partial laryngeal surgery is twice as expensive [66]. This study, however, factored in an average postoperative hospital stay of 4 days for the laser surgery group (approximately 20% of the total cost), which may not be applicable to US practice patterns. In contrast, Cragle and Brandenburg [67] and Brandenburg [68] concluded that the total cost of radiotherapy is much more compared with the cost of laser surgery. Likewise, in a more recent report, Smith and colleagues [69] reported higher actual costs for radiation therapy. Furthermore, these investigators argued that if indirect costs and opportunity costs, such as traveling time, traveling distance, and hours of work missed, are considered, radiation therapy would be associated with higher costs. Overall, one must look at what costs are included and determine whether these are truly relevant in the current practice setting. The best evidence in the United States suggests that there is indeed a cost savings associated with laser surgery for early glottic carcinomas.

Neck management

A retrospective analysis reported that the incidence of occult cervical metastasis in T1 to T2 glottic cancer was 0% [70]. Mendenhall and colleagues [71] looked specifically at T2 glottic squamous cell carcinoma and concluded that cervical lymph nodes are infrequently involved and an elective neck dissection is not warranted. If an issue, however, levels II to IV are at risk for regional metastases. Thus, elective neck dissections are typically not performed in the surgical setting, and prophylactic coverage of the neck is likewise not performed in patients undergoing primary radiation therapy. Watchful waiting with close follow-up is acceptable management for neck metastasis in early-stage glottic cancer.

Summary

The goals of treatment of early glottic cancer are eradication of tumor and preservation of function. Although not supported by a randomized trial, surgery and radiation have comparable rates of local control, ultimate local control, laryngeal preservation, and survival. Tumor factors (eg, involvement of the anterior commissure, location, volume and extent of invasion), patient factors (eg, age, medical comorbidities), and physician and patient preferences after discussion of the indications, risks, benefits, and alternatives should dictate the choice of therapy. Presentation of the cases at a multidisciplinary tumor conference, with representation from the involved specialties to resolve therapeutic conflicts and focus on evidence-based medicine rather than convictions would be beneficial for patients and physicians [72,73].

Regardless of the choice of therapy, smoking cessation, voice therapy, and close surveillance should strongly be encouraged. Rates greater than 20% are reported for second primary malignancies, which are the major cause of death [30,74].

References

[1] Jemal A, Siegel R, Ward E, et al. Cancer statistics, 2007. CA Cancer J Clin 2007;57(1):43–66.
[2] Hoffman HT, Porter K, Karnell LH, et al. Laryngeal cancer in the United States: changes in demographics, patterns of care, and survival. Laryngoscope 2006;116(9 Pt 2 Suppl 111):1–13.
[3] Dey P, Arnold D, Wight R, et al. Radiotherapy versus open surgery versus endolaryngeal surgery (with or without laser) for early laryngeal squamous cell cancer. Cochrane Database Syst Rev 2002;(2):CD002027.
[4] Pfister DG, Laurie SA, Weinstein GS, et al. American Society of Clinical Oncology clinical practice guideline for the use of larynx—preservation strategies in the treatment of laryngeal cancer. J Clin Oncol 2006;24(22):3693–704.
[5] AJCC. AJCC cancer staging manual. 6th edition. New York: Springer; 2002.
[6] Remacle M, Eckel HE, Antonelli A, et al. Endoscopic cordectomy. A proposal for a classification by the Working Committee, European Laryngological Society. Eur Arch Otorhinolaryngol 2000;257(4):227–31.
[7] Remacle M, Van Haverbeke C, Eckel H, et al. Proposal for revision of the European Laryngological Society classification of endoscopic cordectomies. Eur Arch Otorhinolaryngol 2007;264(5):499–504.
[8] Malamou-Mitsi VD, Assimakopoulos DA, Goussia A, et al. Contribution of exfoliative cytology to the diagnosis of laryngeal lesions. Acta Cytol 2000;44(6):993–9.

[9] Moreau PR. Treatment of laryngeal carcinomas by laser endoscopic microsurgery. Laryngoscope 2000;110(6):1000–6.

[10] Ansarin M, Zabrodsky M, Bianchi L, et al. Endoscopic CO2 laser surgery for early glottic cancer in patients who are candidates for radiotherapy: results of a prospective nonrandomized study. Head Neck 2006;28(2):121–5.

[11] Dullerud R, Johansen JG, Dahl T, et al. Influence of CT on tumor classification of laryngeal carcinomas. Acta Radiol 1992;33(4):314–8.

[12] Barbera L, Groome PA, Mackillop WJ, et al. The role of computed tomography in the T classification of laryngeal carcinoma. Cancer 2001;91(2):394–407.

[13] Steiner W. Results of curative laser microsurgery of laryngeal carcinomas. Am J Otolaryngol 1993;14(2):116–21.

[14] Jackel MC, Ambrosch P, Martin A, et al. Impact of re-resection for inadequate margins on the prognosis of upper aerodigestive tract cancer treated by laser microsurgery. Laryngoscope 2007;117(2):350–6.

[15] Eckel HE, Thumfart W, Jungehulsing M, et al. Transoral laser surgery for early glottic carcinoma. Eur Arch Otorhinolaryngol 2000;257(4):221–6.

[16] Spector JG, Sessions DG, Chao KS, et al. Stage I (T1 N0 M0) squamous cell carcinoma of the laryngeal glottis: therapeutic results and voice preservation. Head Neck 1999;21(8):707–17.

[17] Pradhan SA, Pai PS, Neeli SI, et al. Transoral laser surgery for early glottic cancers. Arch Otolaryngol Head Neck Surg 2003;129(6):623–5.

[18] Motta G, Esposito E, Motta S, et al. CO(2) laser surgery in the treatment of glottic cancer. Head Neck 2005;27(7):566–73 [discussion: 573–4].

[19] Rudert HH, Werner JA. Endoscopic resections of glottic and supraglottic carcinomas with the CO2 laser. Eur Arch Otorhinolaryngol 1995;252(3):146–8.

[20] Vilaseca-Gonzalez I, Bernal-Sprekelsen M, Blanch-Alejandro JL, et al. Complications in transoral CO2 laser surgery for carcinoma of the larynx and hypopharynx. Head Neck 2003;25(5):382–8.

[21] Thomas JV, Olsen KD, Neel HB III, et al. Early glottic carcinoma treated with open laryngeal procedures. Arch Otolaryngol Head Neck Surg 1994;120(3):264–8.

[22] Sheen TS, Ko JY, Chang YL. Partial vertical laryngectomy in the treatment of early glottic cancer. Ann Otol Rhinol Laryngol Jul 1998;107(7):593–7.

[23] Giovanni A, Guelfucci B, Gras R, et al. Partial frontolateral laryngectomy with epiglottic reconstruction for management of early-stage glottic carcinoma. Laryngoscope 2001;111(4 Pt 1):663–8.

[24] Laccourreye O, Muscatello L, Laccourreye L, et al. Supracricoid partial laryngectomy with cricohyoidoepiglottopexy for "early" glottic carcinoma classified as T1-T2N0 invading the anterior commissure. Am J Otolaryngol 1997;18(6):385–90.

[25] Spector JG, Sessions DG, Chao KS, et al. Management of stage II (T2N0M0) glottic carcinoma by radiotherapy and conservation surgery. Head Neck 1999;21(2):116–23.

[26] Lee DJ. Definitive radiotherapy for squamous carcinoma of the larynx. Otolaryngol Clin North Am 2002;35(5):1013–33.

[27] Mendenhall WM, Amdur RJ, Morris CG, et al. T1-T2N0 squamous cell carcinoma of the glottic larynx treated with radiation therapy. J Clin Oncol 2001;19(20):4029–36.

[28] Marshak G, Brenner B, Shvero J, et al. Prognostic factors for local control of early glottic cancer: the Rabin Medical Center retrospective study on 207 patients. Int J Radiat Oncol Biol Phys 1999;43(5):1009–13.

[29] Le QT, Fu KK, Kroll S, et al. Influence of fraction size, total dose, and overall time on local control of T1-T2 glottic carcinoma. Int J Radiat Oncol Biol Phys 1997;39(1):115–26.

[30] Cellai E, Frata P, Magrini SM, et al. Radical radiotherapy for early glottic cancer: results in a series of 1087 patients from two Italian radiation oncology centers. I. The case of T1N0 disease. Int J Radiat Oncol Biol Phys 2005;63(5):1378–86.

[31] Warde P, O'Sullivan B, Bristow RG, et al. T1/T2 glottic cancer managed by external beam radiotherapy: the influence of pretreatment hemoglobin on local control. Int J Radiat Oncol Biol Phys 1998;41(2):347–53.

[32] Mendenhall WM, Parsons JT, Million RR, et al. T1-T2 squamous cell carcinoma of the glottic larynx treated with radiation therapy: relationship of dose-fractionation factors to local control and complications. Int J Radiat Oncol Biol Phys 1988;15(6):1267–73.

[33] Johansen LV, Grau C, Overgaard J. Glottic carcinoma—patterns of failure and salvage treatment after curative radiotherapy in 861 consecutive patients. Radiother Oncol 2002; 63(3):257–67.

[34] Frata P, Cellai E, Magrini SM, et al. Radical radiotherapy for early glottic cancer: results in a series of 1087 patients from two Italian radiation oncology centers. II. The case of T2N0 disease. Int J Radiat Oncol Biol Phys 2005;63(5):1387–94.

[35] Garden AS, Forster K, Wong PF, et al. Results of radiotherapy for T2N0 glottic carcinoma: does the "2" stand for twice-daily treatment? Int J Radiat Oncol Biol Phys 2003;55(2): 322–8.

[36] Skladowski K, Tarnawski R, Maciejewski B, et al. Clinical radiobiology of glottic T1 squamous cell carcinoma. Int J Radiat Oncol Biol Phys 1999;43(1):101–6.

[37] Schwaibold F, Scariato A, Nunno M, et al. The effect of fraction size on control of early glottic cancer. Int J Radiat Oncol Biol Phys 1988;14(3):451–4.

[38] Yamazaki H, Nishiyama K, Tanaka E, et al. Radiotherapy for early glottic carcinoma (T1N0M0): results of prospective randomized study of radiation fraction size and overall treatment time. Int J Radiat Oncol Biol Phys 2006;64(1):77–82.

[39] van der Voet JC, Keus RB, Hart AA, et al. The impact of treatment time and smoking on local control and complications in T1 glottic cancer. Int J Radiat Oncol Biol Phys 1998; 42(2):247–55.

[40] Reddy SP, Mohideen N, Marra S, et al. Effect of tumor bulk on local control and survival of patients with T1 glottic cancer. Radiother Oncol 1998;47(2):161–6.

[41] Harwood AR, Hawkins NV, Keane T, et al. Radiotherapy of early glottic cancer. Laryngoscope 1980;90(3):465–70.

[42] Steiner W, Vogt P, Ambrosch P, et al. Transoral carbon dioxide laser microsurgery for recurrent glottic carcinoma after radiotherapy. Head Neck 2004;26(6):477–84.

[43] Rodriguez-Cuevas S, Labastida S, Gonzalez D, et al. Partial laryngectomy as salvage surgery for radiation failures in T1-T2 laryngeal cancer. Head Neck 1998;20(7):630–3.

[44] Schwaab G, Mamelle G, Lartigau E, et al. Surgical salvage treatment of T1/T2 glottic carcinoma after failure of radiotherapy. Am J Surg 1994;168(5):474–5.

[45] Makeieff M, Venegoni D, Mercante G, et al. Supracricoid partial laryngectomies after failure of radiation therapy. Laryngoscope 2005;115(2):353–7.

[46] Ganly I, Patel SG, Matsuo J, et al. Results of surgical salvage after failure of definitive radiation therapy for early-stage squamous cell carcinoma of the glottic larynx. Arch Otolaryngol Head Neck Surg 2006;132(1):59–66.

[47] Ballantyne AJ, Fletcher GH. Surgical management of irradiation failures of nonfixed cancers of the glottic region. Am J Roentgenol Radium Ther Nucl Med 1974;120(1): 164–8.

[48] McLaughlin MP, Parsons JT, Fein DA, et al. Salvage surgery after radiotherapy failure in T1-T2 squamous cell carcinoma of the glottic larynx. Head Neck 1996;18(3):229–35.

[49] Sadri M, McMahon J, Parker A. Management of laryngeal dysplasia: a review. Eur Arch Otorhinolaryngol 2006;263(9):843–52.

[50] Rifai M, Khattab H. Anterior commissure carcinoma: I—histopathologic study. Am J Otolaryngol 2000;21(5):294–7.

[51] Chen MF, Chang JT, Tsang NM, et al. Radiotherapy of early-stage glottic cancer: analysis of factors affecting prognosis. Ann Otol Rhinol Laryngol 2003;112(10):904–11.

[52] Benninger MS, Gillen J, Thieme P, et al. Factors associated with recurrence and voice quality following radiation therapy for T1 and T2 glottic carcinomas. Laryngoscope 1994;104(3 Pt 1): 294–8.

[53] Sombeck MD, Kalbaugh KJ, Mendenhall WM, et al. Radiotherapy for early vocal cord cancer: a dosimetric analysis of 60CO versus 6 MV photons. Head Neck 1996;18(2):167–73.

[54] Steiner W, Ambrosch P, Rodel RM, et al. Impact of anterior commissure involvement on local control of early glottic carcinoma treated by laser microresection. Laryngoscope 2004;114(8):1485–91.

[55] Eckel HE. Local recurrences following transoral laser surgery for early glottic carcinoma: frequency, management, and outcome. Ann Otol Rhinol Laryngol 2001;110(1):7–15.

[56] Bron LP, Soldati D, Zouhair A, et al. Treatment of early stage squamous-cell carcinoma of the glottic larynx: endoscopic surgery or cricohyoidoepiglottopexy versus radiotherapy. Head Neck 2001;23(10):823–9.

[57] Zouhair A, Azria D, Coucke P, et al. Decreased local control following radiation therapy alone in early-stage glottic carcinoma with anterior commissure extension. Strahlenther Onkol 2004;180(2):84–90.

[58] Ledda GP, Grover N, Pundir V, et al. Functional outcomes after CO2 laser treatment of early glottic carcinoma. Laryngoscope 2006;116(6):1007–11.

[59] Casiano RR, Cooper JD, Lundy DS, et al. Laser cordectomy for T1 glottic carcinoma: a 10-year experience and videostroboscopic findings. Otolaryngol Head Neck Surg 1991; 104(6):831–7.

[60] Hirano M, Hirade Y, Kawasaki H. Vocal function following carbon dioxide laser surgery for glottic carcinoma. Ann Otol Rhinol Laryngol 1985;94(3):232–5.

[61] McGuirt WF, Blalock D, Koufman JA, et al. Comparative voice results after laser resection or irradiation of T1 vocal cord carcinoma. Arch Otolaryngol Head Neck Surg 1994;120(9): 951–5.

[62] Cohen SM, Garrett CG, Dupont WD, et al. Voice-related quality of life in T1 glottic cancer: irradiation versus endoscopic excision. Ann Otol Rhinol Laryngol 2006;115(8):581–6.

[63] van Gogh CD, Verdonck-de Leeuw IM, Boon-Kamma BA, et al. The efficacy of voice therapy in patients after treatment for early glottic carcinoma. Cancer 2006;106(1):95–105.

[64] Hocevar-Boltezar I, Zargi M. Voice quality after radiation therapy for early glottic cancer. Arch Otolaryngol Head Neck Surg 2000;126(9):1097–100.

[65] Foote RL, Buskirk SJ, Grado GL, et al. Has radiotherapy become too expensive to be considered a treatment option for early glottic cancer? Head Neck 1997;19(8):692–700.

[66] Gregoire V, Hamoir M, Rosier JF, et al. Cost-minimization analysis of treatment options for T1N0 glottic squamous cell carcinoma: comparison between external radiotherapy, laser microsurgery and partial laryngectomy. Radiother Oncol 1999;53(1):1–13.

[67] Cragle SP, Brandenburg JH. Laser cordectomy or radiotherapy: cure rates, communication, and cost. Otolaryngol Head Neck Surg 1993;108(6):648–54.

[68] Brandenburg JH. Laser cordotomy versus radiotherapy: an objective cost analysis. Ann Otol Rhinol Laryngol 2001;110(4):312–8.

[69] Smith JC, Johnson JT, Cognetti DM, et al. Quality of life, functional outcome, and costs of early glottic cancer. Laryngoscope 2003;113(1):68–76.

[70] Yang CY, Andersen PE, Everts EC, et al. Nodal disease in purely glottic carcinoma: is elective neck treatment worthwhile? Laryngoscope 1998;108(7):1006–8.

[71] Mendenhall WM, Parsons JT, Brant TA, et al. Is elective neck treatment indicated for T2N0 squamous cell carcinoma of the glottic larynx? Radiother Oncol 1989;14(3):199–202.

[72] O'Sullivan B, Mackillop W, Gilbert R, et al. Controversies in the management of laryngeal cancer: results of an international survey of patterns of care. Radiother Oncol 1994;31(1): 23–32.

[73] Goh C, O'Sullivan B, Warde P, et al. Multidisciplinary management controversies in laryngeal cancer. Ann Acad Med Singapore 1996;25(3):405–12.

[74] Franchin G, Minatel E, Gobitti C, et al. Radiotherapy for patients with early-stage glottic carcinoma: univariate and multivariate analyses in a group of consecutive, unselected patients. Cancer 2003;98(4):765–72.

ELSEVIER
SAUNDERS

Otolaryngol Clin N Am
41 (2008) 771–780

OTOLARYNGOLOGIC
CLINICS
OF NORTH AMERICA

Primary and Salvage Total Laryngectomy

Nishant Agrawal, MD[a], David Goldenberg, MD[b],*

[a]Department of Otolaryngology, Head and Neck Surgery, Johns Hopkins University School of
Medicine, 601 North Caroline Street, JHOC 6th Floor, Baltimore, MD 21287, USA
[b]Department of Surgery, Division of Otolaryngology, Head and Neck Surgery, Pennsylvania
State University College of Medicine, PO Box 850,
500 University Drive, MC H091, Hershey, PA 17033, USA

The earliest reference to laryngeal cancer is by Aretaeus in 100 AD. Then Galen, circa 200 AD, described a malignant ulceration of the throat and apparently understood the seriousness of laryngeal cancer. Billroth is credited for performing the first total laryngectomy (TL) for cancer in 1873 [1,2]. Billroth's assistant Carl Gussenbuauer reported this case to the Third Congress of Surgeons.

The results of early laryngectomies were disastrous because of aspiration, pneumonia, hemorrhage, sepsis, mediastinitis, and fistula formation [3]. In 1892, Solis-Cohen devised the principle of suturing the trachea to the skin [4]. Also in the late nineteenth century, Gluck and Soerensen added to the principle of diverting the trachea to the skin and introduced primary reconstruction of the pharynx. Over time, not only has the procedure of TL been modified, but there is also an increasing emphasis on voice and swallowing preservation and/or restoration. In 1980, Singer and Blom [5] introduced the tracheoesophageal puncture (TEP) and valved prosthesis, restoring speech after TL. Eventually, the concept of organ preservation was introduced, and partial laryngeal surgical procedures and chemoradiation protocols became the treatment of choice when possible. Despite these advances, TL still has a role in the treatment of patients who have advanced laryngeal cancer.

Indications

The indications for a TL have decreased as organ preservation strategies have mandated a paradigm shift. In 1991, the Department of Veterans

* Corresponding author.
E-mail address: dgoldenberg@hmc.psu.edu (D. Goldenberg).

0030-6665/08/$ - see front matter © 2008 Elsevier Inc. All rights reserved.
doi:10.1016/j.otc.2008.02.001

Affairs Laryngeal Cancer Study Group demonstrated that induction chemotherapy with cisplatin plus fluorouracil followed by radiation therapy allowed preservation of the larynx in 64% of patients without affecting survival when compared with TL and adjuvant radiotherapy [6]. In 2003, Forastiere and colleagues [7] showed that concurrent chemotherapy with cisplatin and radiotherapy resulted in higher laryngeal preservation rates, better loco-regional control rate, and similar overall survival when compared with induction chemotherapy followed by radiation and radiation therapy alone. In this study, patients who had large-volume T4 disease, defined as tumors with greater than 1 cm invasion of the base of tongue or gross cartilage invasion, were excluded.

Primary TL is indicated in advanced disease that is not amenable to partial laryngectomy, concurrent chemoradiation, or radiotherapy alone. Specifically, tumors that have penetrated through cartilage, invasion into the extralaryngeal soft tissue of the neck, and extensive involvement of the base of tongue are suitable for this procedure. Non-neoplastic indications for primary TL include laryngeal dysfunction with life-threatening aspiration or chondro-radionecrosis of the larynx. Also, pulmonary status and medical comorbidities and cognitive function may define the treatment options for a given patient.

Salvage TL is indicated for chemoradiation, radiation, or partial laryngeal surgical failures. Salvage laryngectomy was required in 16% of patients treated with concurrent chemoradiation and 31% of patients treated with radiotherapy alone [8]. Salvage TL can be technically more difficult and carries a higher postoperative complication rate.

Patient work-up and selection

Beyond the standard history and physical examination, patients must undergo a biopsy to confirm the diagnosis of cancer. Hence, a direct laryngoscopy with biopsy should be performed to help stage the tumor accurately. Esophagoscopy, and bronchoscopy as indicated, should be performed to evaluate for extent of disease and synchronous primary lesions.

A neck CT with contrast also is required in the work-up of advanced laryngeal cancer [9]. A primary indicator for surgery is extensive cartilage invasion. Thyroid cartilage, however, can be either ossified or chondrified, making it difficult to assess erosion by imaging. Yousem and Tufano [10] performed a meta-analysis and reported a sensitivity of 92% and specificity of 79% with MRI of laryngeal infiltration compared with a sensitivity and specificity of 64% and 89%, respectively, with CT. The combination of CT and MRI may be the most effective strategy to evaluate patients who have laryngeal cancer [11]. Furthermore, MRI and/or positron emission tomography (PET) may be useful to diagnose occult neck disease or recurrence [12].

A metastatic screen is also necessary. At the least, this includes a chest radiograph and liver function tests, although these are of uncertain value [13,14]. A chest CT is more effective as a screening tool for pulmonary metastases and second primary tumors [13]. Moreover, often an integrated PET/CT scan may be obtained to evaluate for occult neck or distant metastases, and stage the disease more accurately [15].

The patient must have preoperative clearance to undergo the surgical procedure. Also, the patient is required to have satisfactory performance status/manual dexterity to be able to care for the stoma and TEP prosthesis. Nutritional status and thyroid function should be assessed as well.

Surgical technique

Direct laryngoscopy is performed to determine/confirm the degree of extension of disease and verify the proposed surgical intervention. Modified apron or transverse incision is designed incorporating the existing stoma or planning the permanent stoma. This incision may be modified when performing simultaneous neck dissections.

Subplatysmal flaps are raised to the sternal notch inferiorly, hyoid cartilage superiorly, and sternocleidomastoid muscles laterally. The sternocleidomastoid muscles are exposed. The strap muscles are transected 1 cm above the clavicle and elevated from the laryngotracheal complex. The thyroid isthmus is divided; the ipsilateral thyroid gland and paratracheal lymph nodes typically are taken with the specimen, especially when there is extralaryngeal disease or subglottic spread. The contralateral thyroid lobe is freed from the trachea and mobilized laterally.

The superior boarder of the hyoid cartilage is freed by transecting the suprahyoid musculature. The greater cornu are skeletonized carefully so as not to jeopardize the hypoglossal nerve and lingual artery. The larynx is rotated, and the posterior border of the thyroid cartilage is skeletonized by separating the laryngeal constrictors. Bilateral inferior cornus and superior cornus are skeletonized. The superior laryngeal neurovascular structures are divided. The pyriform sinus mucosa is dissected away from the inner thyroid cartilage lamina if oncologically appropriate.

Once the laryngotracheal complex is mobilized, horizontal tracheal cuts are made at a level at least 1 cm beyond the tumor. The trachea is entered, and an endotracheal tube is placed in the trachea. The anterior tracheal cuts are beveled superiorly, and the posterior wall tracheal cut is placed more cephalad. This provides a larger area for the stoma. The posterior trachea wall then is separated from the cervical esophagus.

A pharyngotomy may be made through the contralateral pyriform sinus or by means of the vallecula. Under direct visualization of the mucosal surfaces, the larynx is resected free taking care to preserve adequate uninvolved mucosa for closure. Frozen section margins should be analyzed.

A cricopharyngeal myotomy is performed by sharply dividing the circumferential muscle bands up to the serosal layer.

If a TEP is planned, it is performed at this point. Primary TEP is placed through the common posterior wall, 1 cm below the posterior wall of the free end of the trachea. A temporary catheter or prosthesis is placed to stent the tract.

The pharyngeal mucosa is closed using a running inverting suture. This may be done in a T, vertical, or horizontal fashion [16]. The closure should be tension-free. The suture line can be reinforced with a second imbricating suture line if necessary.

Sofferman and Voronetsky [17] describe the use of a linear stapler for pharyngoesophageal closure after TL. A bougie may be placed, and a gastrointestinal TA 60 stapler is used to separate the larynx and close the pharynx.

Drains are placed in the neopharynx gutter on each side and secured. The tracheal stoma is matured by suturing the end of the trachea to the skin in an interrupted fashion with half vertical mattress sutures. The skin then is closed in layers.

Postoperatively, routine care is instituted, including wound care, stoma care, drain care, fluid management, and pain management. Nutritional status and thyroid function should be optimized.

Neck

The larynx drains into levels 2 to 4 pretracheal and paratracheal lymph nodes within the neck. Advanced laryngeal cancers have an overall 30% incidence of occult neck metastasis [18]. Patients who have supraglottic and advanced glottic with clinically N0 neck should undergo elective treatment of the neck by either neck dissection or radiotherapy [19]. Supraglottic tumors have a significant propensity for bilateral neck metastasis, and bilateral necks should be addressed [20]. Patients with N1 disease who are treated with definitive chemoradiotherapy require a neck dissection for incomplete clinical response [21]. Neck dissection arguably is required for patients with N2 or N3 disease who are treated with definitive chemoradiotherapy [21–23]. For salvage surgery, the decision to perform a neck dissection should be based on CT staging of the neck, as most patients who are radiologically staged N0 are unlikely to harbor occult nodal disease [24].

Adjuvant radiation

Adjuvant radiotherapy may be combined with primary TL for advanced laryngeal carcinomas. The goal of adjuvant radiotherapy is to control locoregional minimal residual disease. More specifically, postoperative radiation therapy is indicated in patients with T4 carcinoma, inadequate surgical margins, cervical lymph nodes metastasis, and extracapsular, perineural, and/or vascular spread [25–28]. Nevertheless, Spector and colleagues [29] did not demonstrate a statistically significant difference in recurrence or disease-specific survival with TL alone compared with combined TL and radiotherapy. Likewise, Cortesina and colleagues [28] reported comparable survival in patients who underwent surgery only and combined therapy, but the latter group was comprised of patients who had more negative prognostic factors. Hence, they concluded radiotherapy was effective in controlling minimal residual disease.

Complications

Early complications after TL include bleeding/hematoma, infection, wound breakdown, and pharyngocutaneous fistula formation. In the case of bleeding, the patient should be explored in the operating room with evacuation of the clot and control of bleeding. A wound infection is managed by opening the wound and draining the infected collection, followed by packing and culture-specific antibiotics.

Pharyngocutaneous fistula is a common, troublesome complication. The incidence is generally higher after combination treatment, approximating 20% to 30% in patients treated with radiotherapy or concomitant chemoradiotherapy [8,30]. Ganly and colleagues [31] showed that chemoradiotherapy was an independent predictor of pharyngocutaneous fistula formation. In a meta-analysis, preoperative radiotherapy was associated with increased relative risk of pharyngocutaneous fistula [32]. Furthermore, the study suggested irradiated patients had increased duration and severity of the fistula. Pharyngocutaneous fistula is treated conservatively with maintaining the patient nothing by mouth, wound packing, and antibiotics. A biopsy may be indicated to exclude persistent/recurrent cancer. If conservative management is unsuccessful after a few weeks, operative intervention with a vascularized flap is considered. If the carotid arteries are exposed, flap coverage is necessary to avoid the sometimes fatal outcomes of a carotid erosion and bleed. In fact, Withrow and colleagues [33] claimed that prophylactic reconstruction with a vascularized flap after a salvage laryngectomy was associated with a lower fistula rate of 18% versus 50% for primary closure. Fung and colleagues [34], however, reported that vascularized tissue did not reduce the fistula rate in salvage laryngectomy patients, although the severity was less when compared with patients who underwent primary closure.

Late complications include stomal stenosis, pharyngoesophageal stricture/stenosis, and hypothyroidism. Stomal stenosis can be managed with a stomal button/laryngectomy tube or stomaplasty. The most effective means to treat stomal stenosis, however, is prevention with proper surgical technique during the laryngectomy. Pharyngoesophageal stenosis can be treated with dilation. In this situation, recurrence/persistence of cancer may need to be ruled out. Hypothyroidism is a relatively common occurrence, especially after combination therapy with radiation and laryngectomy [35]. Thyroid function tests should be periodically checked postoperatively/after radiation, and thyroid replacement hormone should be initiated as needed [36].

Recurrence

In a recent study, approximately 31% of patients who underwent a TL for primary tumor or for salvage therapy had recurrence, defined as loco-regional recurrence, second primaries, or distant metastases [37]. The mean interval between TL and detection of recurrence was 11.6 months. Almost 60% of patients had loco-regional recurrence, most commonly in the neck or tracheostomal recurrence. Approximately 25% had metastatic disease, and most of the remaining patients had a second primary malignancy.

Tracheostomal recurrence after TL typically carries a dismal prognosis. The incidence of stomal recurrence ranges between 3% and 15% [37–42]. Factors that predispose to stomal recurrence include subglottic extension to greater than 1 cm, inadequate margins of tracheal resection, and paratracheal lymph node involvement. Treatment options are limited but include aggressive surgery [43], radiotherapy, or chemotherapy.

Swallowing

Intraoperatively, either a nasogastric tube or a temporary catheter is placed in the tracheoesophageal fistula. Tube feeds are begun once bowel sounds are present. Common practice is to initiate oral feeding on postoperative day 5 to 7 in nonradiated patients, and 7 to 14 postoperative days in radiated patients. There is evidence, however, that oral feeding may be commenced on postoperative days 2 to 3 without increasing the rate of a fistula [44,45].

Dysphagia warrants a modified barium swallow study to evaluate for anatomic abnormalities. Dilation of the stenotic segment may be performed if structural narrowing is evident on videofluoroscopic imaging. Pseudoepiglottis, more common with vertical closures, is treated with dietary modification or surgical removal [46]. Behavioral changes and postural changes are also helpful maneuvers to improve swallowing dysfunction.

Voice

The three methods of communication after a TL include TEP speech, esophageal speech, and artificial or mechanical larynx. Today, tracheoesophageal speech is the preferred form of voice rehabilitation after TL [47,48]. Tracheoesophageal speech functions by forcing air through a one-way valve into a narrow pharyngoesophageal segment that vibrates to produce sound. To achieve intelligible speech and successful voice rehabilitation, patients are encouraged to work closely with the speech pathologists pre- and postoperatively.

TEP may be performed either primarily or secondarily. The basic procedure of a primary TEP has been described. Several variations exist for secondary TEP, including the one described by Koch [49].

A voice prosthesis is placed within the surgically produced fistula and acts as a one- way valve, allowing passage of air from the trachea into the esophagus, while preventing aspiration and maintaining the tract. This can be done at the time of surgery or 1 to 2 weeks after surgery, but voicing should be delayed until healing of the pharyngotomy closure is complete. Hands-free speech may be accomplished by using a specialized stoma valve [50].

Common problems following TEP include failure of voice restoration, leakage around or through the prosthesis, and granulation tissue formation. Fortunately, more serious complications occur infrequently. Speech acquisition rates range from 58% to 93% [51,52]. Common causes of failure to achieve speech include patient factors, poor prosthesis fit, and pharyngoesophageal spasm, stricture, or hypotonicity. Fluoroscopy is helpful to differentiate the different pharyngoesophageal conditions. Pharyngoesophageal spasm/hypertonicity, the most common cause of failure, can be treated with behavioral modification, botulinum toxin, myotomy, or neurectomy [53–57]. Pharyngoesophageal stricture generally is treated with dilation, but may require open pharyngoplasty and flap reconstruction. Hypotonicity can be treated by application of pressure above the stoma to narrow the pharyngeal walls to facilitate voice production.

Leakage can be caused either by prosthesis failure or enlargement of the tracheoesophageal fistula. The valves must be maintained and kept clean to ensure proper functioning. A common cause of device failure is yeast colonization, which can be treated with oral antifungals [58]. An enlarged tracheoesophageal fistula may be addressed by temporary placement of a catheter in place of the prosthesis to allow the fistula to contract. Surgical repair, or even closure of the fistula, may be required to prevent aspiration and its sequelae. Granulation tissue is treated with replacement of the prosthesis and silver nitrate cauterization.

Summary

TL continues to play a major role in the treatment of advanced laryngeal cancer or for recurrent/persistent disease after failed organ preservation attempts. Functional rehabilitation is available, and most patients are able to communicate effectively with tracheoesophageal speech and maintain swallowing function.

References

[1] Absolon KB, Keshishian J. First laryngectomy for cancer as performed by Theodor Billroth on December 31, 1873: a hundred anniversary. Rev Surg 1974;31(2):65–70.

[2] Weir NF. Theodore Billroth: the first laryngectomy for cancer. J Laryngol Otol 1973;87(12): 1161–9.

[3] Genden EM, Ferlito A, Silver CE, et al. Evolution of the management of laryngeal cancer. Oral Oncol 2007;43(5):431–9.

[4] Ferlito A, Silver CE, Zeitels SM, et al. Evolution of laryngeal cancer surgery. Acta Otolaryngol 2002;122(6):665–72.

[5] Singer MI, Blom ED. An endoscopic technique for restoration of voice after laryngectomy. Ann Otol Rhinol Laryngol 1980;89(6 Pt 1):529–33.

[6] Induction chemotherapy plus radiation compared with surgery plus radiation in patients with advanced laryngeal cancer. The Department of Veterans Affairs Laryngeal Cancer Study Group. N Engl J Med 1991;324(24):1685–90.

[7] Forastiere AA, Goepfert H, Maor M, et al. Concurrent chemotherapy and radiotherapy for organ preservation in advanced laryngeal cancer. N Engl J Med 2003;349(22):2091–8.

[8] Weber RS, Berkey BA, Forastiere A, et al. Outcome of salvage total laryngectomy following organ preservation therapy: the Radiation Therapy Oncology Group trial 91–11. Arch Otolaryngol Head Neck Surg 2003;129(1):44–9.

[9] Dullerud R, Johansen JG, Dahl T, et al. Influence of CT on tumor classification of laryngeal carcinomas. Acta Radiol 1992;33(4):314–8.

[10] Yousem DM, Tufano RP. Laryngeal imaging. Neuroimaging Clin N Am 2004;14(4):611–24.

[11] Becker M. (Diagnosis and staging of laryngeal tumors with CT and MRI). Radiologe 1998; 38(2):93–100 [in German].

[12] Terhaard CH, Bongers V, van Rijk PP, et al. F-18-fluoro-deoxy-glucose positron emission tomography scanning in detection of local recurrence after radiotherapy for laryngeal/pharyngeal cancer. Head Neck 2001;23(11):933–41.

[13] Houghton DJ, Hughes ML, Garvey C, et al. Role of chest CT scanning in the management of patients presenting with head and neck cancer. Head Neck 1998;20(7):614–8.

[14] Korver KD, Graham SM, Hoffman HT, et al. Liver function studies in the assessment of head and neck cancer patients. Head Neck 1995;17(6):531–4.

[15] Schwartz DL, Rajendran J, Yueh B, et al. Staging of head and neck squamous cell cancer with extended-field FDG-PET. Arch Otolaryngol Head Neck Surg 2003;129(11):1173–8.

[16] Bedrin L, Ginsburg G, Horowitz Z, et al. 25-year experience of using a linear stapler in laryngectomy. Head Neck 2005;27(12):1073–9.

[17] Sofferman RA, Voronetsky I. Use of the linear stapler for pharyngoesophageal closure after total laryngectomy. Laryngoscope 2000;110(8):1406–9.

[18] Kligerman J, Olivatto LO, Lima RA, et al. Elective neck dissection in the treatment of T3/T4 N0 squamous cell carcinoma of the larynx. Am J Surg 1995;170(5):436–9.

[19] Redaelli de Zinis LO, Nicolai P, Tomenzoli D, et al. The distribution of lymph node metastases in supraglottic squamous cell carcinoma: therapeutic implications. Head Neck 2002; 24(10):913–20.

[20] Lutz CK, Johnson JT, Wagner RL, et al. Supraglottic carcinoma: patterns of recurrence. Ann Otol Rhinol Laryngol 1990;99(1):12–7.

[21] Pfister DG, Laurie SA, Weinstein GS, et al. American Society of Clinical Oncology clinical practice guideline for the use of larynx-preservation strategies in the treatment of laryngeal cancer. J Clin Oncol 2006;24(22):3693–704.

[22] McHam SA, Adelstein DJ, Rybicki LA, et al. Who merits a neck dissection after definitive chemoradiotherapy for N2-N3 squamous cell head and neck cancer? Head Neck 2003; 25(10):791–8.

[23] Brizel DM, Prosnitz RG, Hunter S, et al. Necessity for adjuvant neck dissection in setting of concurrent chemoradiation for advanced head and neck cancer. Int J Radiat Oncol Biol Phys 2004;58(5):1418–23.

[24] Farrag TY, Lin FR, Cummings CW, et al. Neck management in patients undergoing post-radiotherapy salvage laryngeal surgery for recurrent/persistent laryngeal cancer. Laryngoscope 2006;116(10):1864–6.

[25] Jesse RH. The evaluation of treatment of patients with extensive squamous cancer of the vocal cords. Laryngoscope 1975;85(9):1424–9.

[26] Yuen A, Medina JE, Goepfert H, et al. Management of stage T3 and T4 glottic carcinomas. Am J Surg 1984;148(4):467–72.

[27] De Stefani A, Magnano M, Cavalot A, et al. Adjuvant radiotherapy influences the survival of patients with squamous carcinoma of the head and neck who have poor prognoses. Otolaryngol Head Neck Surg 2000;123(5):630–6.

[28] Cortesina G, De Stefani A, Cavalot A, et al. Current role of radiotherapy in the treatment of locally advanced laryngeal carcinomas. J Surg Oncol 2000;74(1):79–82.

[29] Spector GJ, Sessions DG, Lenox J, et al. Management of stage IV glottic carcinoma: therapeutic outcomes. Laryngoscope 2004;114(8):1438–46.

[30] Grau C, Johansen LV, Hansen HS, et al. Salvage laryngectomy and pharyngocutaneous fistulae after primary radiotherapy for head and neck cancer: a national survey from DAHANCA. Head Neck 2003;25(9):711–6.

[31] Ganly I, Patel S, Matsuo J, et al. Postoperative complications of salvage total laryngectomy. Cancer 2005;103(10):2073–81.

[32] Paydarfar JA, Birkmeyer NJ. Complications in head and neck surgery: a meta-analysis of postlaryngectomy pharyngocutaneous fistula. Arch Otolaryngol Head Neck Surg 2006; 132(1):67–72.

[33] Withrow KP, Rosenthal EL, Gourin CG, et al. Free tissue transfer to manage salvage laryngectomy defects after organ preservation failure. Laryngoscope 2007;117(5):781–4.

[34] Fung K, Teknos TN, Vandenberg CD, et al. Prevention of wound complications following salvage laryngectomy using free vascularized tissue. Head Neck 2007;29(5):425–30.

[35] Leon X, Gras JR, Perez A, et al. Hypothyroidism in patients treated with total laryngectomy. A multivariate study. Eur Arch Otorhinolaryngol 2002;259(4):193–6.

[36] Smolarz K, Malke G, Voth E, et al. Hypothyroidism after therapy for larynx and pharynx carcinoma. Thyroid 2000;10(5):425–9.

[37] Ritoe SC, Bergman H, Krabbe PF, et al. Cancer recurrence after total laryngectomy: treatment options, survival, and complications. Head Neck 2006;28(5):383–8.

[38] Imauchi Y, Ito K, Takasago E, et al. Stomal recurrence after total laryngectomy for squamous cell carcinoma of the larynx. Otolaryngol Head Neck Surg 2002;126(1):63–6.

[39] Zbaren P, Greiner R, Kengelbacher M. Stoma recurrence after laryngectomy: an analysis of risk factors. Otolaryngol Head Neck Surg 1996;114(4):569–75.

[40] Rubin J, Johnson JT, Myers EN. Stomal recurrence after laryngectomy: interrelated risk factor study. Otolaryngol Head Neck Surg 1990;103(5 Pt 1):805–12.

[41] Mantravadi R, Katz AM, Skolnik EM, et al. Stomal recurrence. A critical analysis of risk factors. Arch Otolaryngol 1981;107(12):735–8.

[42] Weber RS, Marvel J, Smith P, et al. Paratracheal lymph node dissection for carcinoma of the larynx, hypopharynx, and cervical esophagus. Otolaryngol Head Neck Surg 1993;108(1): 11–7.

[43] Gluckman JL, Hamaker RC, Schuller DE, et al. Surgical salvage for stomal recurrence: a multi-institutional experience. Laryngoscope 1987;97(9):1025–9.

[44] Aprigliano F. Use of the nasogastric tube after total laryngectomy: is it truly necessary? Ann Otol Rhinol Laryngol 1990;99(7 Pt 1):513–4.

[45] Medina JE, Khafif A. Early oral feeding following total laryngectomy. Laryngoscope 2001; 111(3):368–72.

[46] Davis RK, Vincent ME, Shapshay SM, et al. The anatomy and complications of "T" versus vertical closure of the hypopharynx after laryngectomy. Laryngoscope 1982;92(1):16–22.

[47] Williams SE, Watson JB. Speaking proficiency variations according to method of laryngeal voicing. Laryngoscope 1987;97(6):737–9.

[48] Clements KS, Rassekh CH, Seikaly H, et al. Communication after laryngectomy. An assessment of patient satisfaction. Arch Otolaryngol Head Neck Surg 1997;123(5):493–6.

[49] Koch WM. A failsafe technique for endoscopic tracheoesophageal puncture. Laryngoscope 2001;111(9):1663–5.

[50] Blom ED, Singer MI, Hamaker RC. Tracheostoma valve for postlaryngectomy voice rehabilitation. Ann Otol Rhinol Laryngol 1982;91(6 Pt 1):576–8.

[51] Kao WW, Mohr RM, Kimmel CA, et al. The outcome and techniques of primary and secondary tracheoesophageal puncture. Arch Otolaryngol Head Neck Surg 1994;120(3):301–7.

[52] Lau WF, Wei WI, Ho CM, et al. Immediate tracheoesophageal puncture for voice restoration in laryngopharyngeal resection. Am J Surg 1988;156(4):269–72.

[53] Blitzer A, Komisar A, Baredes S, et al. Voice failure after tracheoesophageal puncture: management with botulinum toxin. Otolaryngol Head Neck Surg 1995;113(6):668–70.

[54] Lewin JS, Bishop-Leone JK, Forman AD, et al. Further experience with Botox injection for tracheoesophageal speech failure. Head Neck 2001;23(6):456–60.

[55] Singer MI, Blom ED, Hamaker RC. Pharyngeal plexus neurectomy for laryngeal speech rehabilitation. Laryngoscope 1986;96(1):50–4.

[56] Singer MI, Blom ED. Selective myotomy for voice restoration after total laryngectomy. Arch Otolaryngol 1981;107(11):670–3.

[57] Crary MA, Glowasky AL. Using botulinum toxin A to improve speech and swallowing function following total laryngectomy. Arch Otolaryngol Head Neck Surg 1996;122(7):760–3.

[58] Leder SB, Erskine MC. Voice restoration after laryngectomy: experience with the Blom-Singer extended-wear indwelling tracheoesophageal voice prosthesis. Head Neck 1997; 19(6):487–93.

ELSEVIER
SAUNDERS

Otolaryngol Clin N Am
41 (2008) 781–791

OTOLARYNGOLOGIC
CLINICS
OF NORTH AMERICA

Applications of Robotics
for Laryngeal Surgery

Alexander T. Hillel, MD[a], Ankur Kapoor, PhD[b],
Nabil Simaan, PhD[c], Russell H. Taylor, PhD[d],
Paul Flint, MD[a],*

[a]*Department of Otolaryngology, Head and Neck Surgery, Johns Hopkins
University School of Medicine, 601 N. Caroline Street, 6th Floor, JHOC 6163,
Baltimore, MD 21287-0910, USA*
[b]*National Institutes of Health, Bethesda Clinical Center, 9000 Rockville Pike,
Bethesda, MD 20892, USA*
[c]*Department of Mechanical Engineering, Columbia University, 234 S.W. Mudd,
Mail Code: 4703 500 West 120th Street, New York, NY 10027, USA*
[d]*Department of Computer Science, Whiting School of Engineering, Johns Hopkins University
CSEB 127, 3400 N. Charles Street, Baltimore, MD 21218, USA*

The anatomy of the upper airway lends difficulty to the surgical treatment of laryngeal disease. Open surgery of the larynx allows for increased exposure of the surgical field and dexterity of instrumentation; however, healthy tissue, especially the delicate vibratory tissues and framework of the larynx, may be damaged during the procedure. In contrast, endoscopic laryngeal surgery uses natural body openings and therefore minimizes resultant damage to the framework. Even with advancements over the past 30 years, endoscopic laryngeal surgery continues to have disadvantages, including the operator's distance from the surgical field, the laryngoscope's relatively small exposure, and reduced depth perception with binocular vision. The lack of steerable modular instrumentation and three-dimensional (3D) viewing further handicap the laryngologist's distal dexterity and suturing ability [1]. Minimally invasive robotic surgery has the potential to address the shortcomings of endolaryngeal surgery and to significantly advance laryngeal surgery.

Endoscopic laryngeal surgery reduced invasiveness and improved outcomes since its introduction almost 100 years ago. In 1915, Lynch [2] first

* Corresponding author.
E-mail address: pflint@jhmi.edu (P. Flint).

reported the use of a laryngoscope for excision of glottic cancer. Lynch's use of suspension laryngoscopy allowed for bimanual operation of instruments. Four decades later, Rosemarie Albrecht reported the addition of microscopy to enhance visualization of the larynx [3]. Jako [4] and Kleinsasser [5] further refined laryngeal microsurgery by providing depth perception with binocular vision. Instrumentation evolved along with this new operative approach as microlaryngeal scissors, graspers, grippers, mirrors, elevators and suction devices were designed. The next development arrived in the early 1970s, when Jako and Strong [6,7] combined the carbon dioxide laser with the operating microscope to provide for precise cutting and cauterization. Since then, lasers have been further refined with the microspot laser and microlaryngeal instruments have been further miniaturized. The powered microdebrider has been added to the armamentarium to lessen the operative time of and thermal damage caused by the laser [8,9].

Other than miniaturization and the introduction of a few powered instruments, endolaryngeal surgery has evolved little in the past 30 years. The typical operative arrays employ either a handheld endoscope with one free hand to manipulate an instrument or the use of a binocular microscope that provides two hands to manipulate instruments (Fig. 1). With either arrangement, the laryngoscope predetermines the port of instrument entry and provides a confined space that leads to instrument collision and often an obstructed view (Fig. 2). Laryngologists remain restricted by the operator's distance from the surgical field, the laryngoscope's relatively small exposure, and reduced depth perception with binocular vision. These combine to restrict the surgeon's ability to manipulate instruments across the long distance from the oral cavity to the larynx, resulting in poor sensory feedback (both visual and tactile) and magnification of operator tremor.

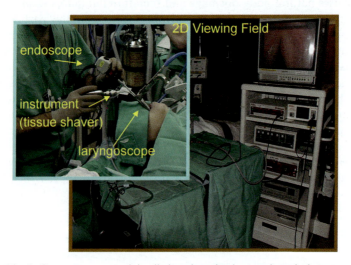

Fig. 1. Common current minimally invasive microlaryngeal surgical set-up.

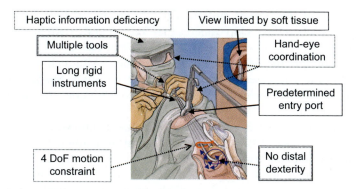

Fig. 2. Limitations of typical minimally invasive surgery (*dashed lines*) and current microlar-yngeal (*solid lines*) surgery.

Additionally, the lack of distal dexterity often causes damage to surrounding healthy tissue and limits surgical wound healing. While Woo and colleagues established endolaryngeal suturing techniques, suture repair of vocal fold wounds remains challenging due to technical complexities and the resulting increase in operative time [10]. Suturing limitations result in larger scar formation. Fleming and colleagues [11] demonstrated a 75% larger scar area when laryngeal defects healed with secondary intention versus primary intention. Larger vocal fold scars translate into worse voice outcomes. At this time, endoscopic laryngeal surgery has reached an impasse as the lack of distal instrument mobility, complexity of suture technique, and poor 3D vision limit surgical techniques that are routine in other surgical subspecialties.

Robotic equipment for laryngeal surgery has the potential to overcome many of the limitations of endolaryngeal procedures by improving optics, increasing instrument degrees of freedom, and modulating tremor. Currently, robotic surgery is employed in various specialties and in some cases has become the preferred procedure. The most commonly used system is the da Vinci Surgical Robot (Intuitive Surgical Inc, Sunnyvale, California), which is available at more than 170 hospitals throughout the United States [12]. The da Vinci system was approved by the Food and Drug Administration (FDA) for general laparoscopic surgery in 2000 and thoracoscopy in 2001 [13]. Robotic surgery has been employed in urologic surgery [14] and gynecologic surgery, as well as to perform cardiac valve repair and coronary artery bypass grafting [15,16]. The da Vinci Surgical Robot incorporates independently steerable arms and 3D imaging into a surgical cart and surgeon's console. The surgeon's console provides control of instrument arms with master robot manipulators. The surgical cart contains the slave robotic manipulators consisting of three arms: one to handle the endoscopic camera with the other two arms holding either two 8-mm (conventional adult size) or two 5-mm (pediatric size) endowrist instruments with increased distal freedom of motion. The 12-mm stereoscopic endoscope is equipped with two three-chip cameras that feed separate right and left views back to the vision cart, which creates a 3D perspective for the surgeon with separate monitors for right eye and left eye vision. Although its optics and tremor filtration represent key advances, the da Vinci Surgical Robot's freedom of motion provides the greatest contribution to the surgical armamentarium.

The human arm represents the greatest actuator known to humans and represents the basis for which robotic surgical manipulators are constructed. The human arm is considered to have seven degrees of freedom provided by three joints. Degrees of freedom (DoF) are often described using nautical terminology such as pitch (tilting in a vertical vector), yaw (turning to the left or right), and roll (tilting from side to side). The shoulder is capable of pitch, yaw, and roll, the elbow pitch, and the wrist pitch, yaw and roll, totaling seven DoF. The elbow actuator of the human arm breaks the connection between the shoulder and wrist allowing for roll at both joints. That differs substantially from an endolaryngeal instrument being manipulated by a human arm or the da Vinci surgical robot effector arm. Endolaryngeal instruments are limited by their straight shaft, lack of a wrist actuator, and the small opening of the laryngoscope. When operated by the human hand, endolaryngeal instruments have four DoF: the yaw, pitch, and roll of the human hand and the ability to move in an out. The degrees of yaw and pitch are limited by the laryngoscope's opening. When compared with the human arm, the da Vinci surgical robot has six DoF. The unique isocenter of motion-proximal actuator allows each robotic arm to pivot around a point outside of the volume of the actuator. That is usually at the point of insertion into the human body, which would be the equivalent of the shoulder in a human arm analogy. However, because the robotic arm is a straight shaft (lacking the elbow of the human arm), the roll at the point of skin insertion is the same roll at the endowrist joint. Therefore, the six DoF of each da Vinci slave manipulator are from yaw and pitch at the endowrist and skin insertion point, roll along the shaft, and the ability to move in and out of the port. These six DoF allow for comparable tissue manipulation to that of the human arm during open surgical procedures and its application has the potential to greatly advance laryngeal surgery.

The enthusiasm for applications of robotic surgery in otolaryngology–head and neck surgery have been slowed by ease of access to body orifices and the relative ease of hiding surgical wounds out of the line of site in the hairline or in mucous membranes. Applications in laryngeal robotic surgery have been further limited by the endotracheal tube in the operative field and manipulation of the robotic instrument arms in the narrow oral, pharyngeal, and laryngeal spaces [17]. Furthermore, the da Vinci Surgical Robot was designed for opposing arms inserted via widely spaced ports of entry in the abdomen and thorax. These applications are quite different from the need for parallel ports of entry through the narrow opening of a laryngoscope.

In 2005, McLeod and Melder [18] were the first to report use of the da Vinci Surgical Robot in laryngeal surgery, performing a robotic-assisted excision of a vallecular cyst. The authors used a slotted laryngoscope, which only provided operative space for one 8-mm robotic arm in addition to the 12-mm stereoscopic camera. A surgeon assisted on the case by providing olive tip tissue countertraction. The robot's arm successfully marsupialized the cyst with round-tip cautery, procured biopsies of the cyst wall, and placed oxymetazoline-soaked pledgets for hemostasis. The procedure was performed without complication and the patient was discharged the same day. The total case time was 109 minutes, however 89 minutes were spent setting up the robot. The authors concluded that superb 3D visualization allowed for accurate assessment and precise instrument control [18]. While it was feasible to use the robot in the human airway, the laryngoscope provided limited space for operative maneuvering.

The volume limitations of the laryngoscope were overcome with the use of a mouth gag to retract the mouth tongue and cheeks. Hockstein and colleagues [17,19] reported the technical feasibility of operating with the three arms of the da Vinci Surgical Robot through a Dingman mouth gag for airway surgery on a mannequin and cadavers. The Dingman mouth gag with cheek retractors achieved satisfactory exposure, unimpeded instrument movement, precise handling of tissue, and an ability to perform endolaryngeal suturing. Initial experiments focused on various pharyngeal and microlaryngeal procedures, including arytenoidectomy, partial epiglottectomy, and partial resection of the base of tongue to demonstrate efficacy with the robot. In each procedure the tongue was retracted, a 30-degree upward-facing endoscope was used for visualization, and both 5-mm and 8-mm diameter instruments were used. The duration of each procedure was comparable to conventional operative methods. Furthermore, Hockstein and colleagues [19] reported an increase in freedom of instrument mobility, improved depth perception with the 3D imaging, scaling of movement (from the large movement of the operator's hand to the small movement of instrument), and removal of tremor. Last, Hockstein and colleagues [20] concluded that the safety profile of transoral robotic surgery was comparable to that of conventional endoscopic laryngeal surgery.

Success with cadaveric robotic surgery has translated into clinical experimentation with the da Vinci Surgical Robot, including published reports of transoral robotic supraglottic partial laryngectomy and base of tongue neoplasm resection [12,21–23]. Preclinical studies animal studies preceded each clinical study of three patients [21,23]. Both studies used 8-mm instrumentation with visualization by 0° and 30° high magnification endoscopes through FK mouth retractors. These studies introduced the use of electrocautery robotic instruments and a flexible tracheal suction device manipulated by a robotic arm [12,22]. A surgeon assisted each robotic procedure with the application of surgical clips. The mean surgical time for supraglottic transoral robotic surgery was 120 minutes, while the base of tongue procedures averaged 105 minutes [12]. These results included robotic positioning and exposure, however the results omitted set-up time. The six procedures in both studies were completed robotically without complication and with minimal blood loss [12,22]. The authors concluded that base of tongue neoplasm excision and supraglottic laryngectomy were technically feasible and safe with the da Vinci Surgical Robot, allowing for good exposure and complete tumor resection.

In a separate study, Rahbar and colleagues [24] described success using the da Vinci Surgical Robot in pediatric airway surgery to repair laryngeal clefts in five patients. Before the introduction of the robot, a carbon dioxide laser was used to denude the mucosal margin of the cleft. A Crowe-Davis mouth gag provided sufficient exposure to employ both a 0° and 30° endoscope, with the 30° endoscope providing superior exposure of the glottis. The authors described restricted movement with both 5-mm and 8-mm-diameter instruments. Ultimately, inadequate surgical access resulted in abandoning the robotic approach in three patients. In the other two patients, transoral robotic repair was successful as defined by endolaryngeal suturing to close the cleft [24]. In these cases, robotic operative time was increased by an average of 40 minutes as compared with routine endoscopic approach [24].

Robotic surgery has clear advantages in motor control and visualization when compared with conventional endoscopic laryngeal surgery. The da Vinci Surgical Robot's 3D optics system creates a superb wide-view high-definition illusion of a 3D surgical field. Its movable endoscope expands the surgical field by changing viewing angles and position translating to greater surgical precision. Motor control is improved with a combination of movement scaling, tremor modulation, and increased instrument freedom of motion. The da Vinci master-slave robotic manipulators filter out natural hand tremor, adjust the large hand movements of the operator to the small movements of instruments in the airway, and enhance dexterity, to allow for more precise instrument movement and prevent instrument collision within the airway [24–26]. Instrument control is further enhanced with distal articulation by the da Vinci's endowrist design, providing flexion, extension, pronation, and supination at the distal end of instruments for finer tissue manipulation.

In comparison to transoral laser surgery, robotic surgery's rotational optics is superior to line-of-sight visualization with the operating microscope. Furthermore, the robotic arms allow for en bloc tumor resection as opposed to the piecemeal cutting of the tumor with the laser [22]. Finally, robotic airway surgery allows for certain procedures that are more commonly performed with an open approach, such as excision of supraglottic or base of tongue cancer, to be successfully completed through an endoscope. This decreases morbidity to adjacent tissue and bony structures associated with open procedures and precludes need for tracheostomy [22].

While the da Vinci Surgical Robot has advantages over open and endoscopic laryngeal surgery, there are limitations in its design. The current da Vinci robot was designed for abdominal and thoracic surgery with large-diameter instruments predicated on laparoscopic instruments. The arms of the robot were designed to mimic the opposition of a surgeon's hands in conventional surgery; the robot arms were not designed to be coaxial with the lumen of a laryngoscope. The current 12-mm-diameter endoscope competes with space with 8-mm adult and 5-mm pediatric instruments. This is evidenced by McLeod and Melder's [18] inability to place both robotic arms within the laryngoscope during their robot-assisted excision of a vallecular cyst. They also reported a lengthy set-up process that took two-and-a-half times as long as the procedure itself [18]. Last, their robot arms did not have a suction device, which was provided by a surgeon-assistant [18]. While Weinstein and colleagues ultimately attached an endotracheal suction to a robotic arm, the current da Vinci robot lacks an integrated suction device [12]. While all three robotic arms fit through the mouth gag, both Hockstein and colleagues [17] and Rahbar and colleagues [24] reported limited access resulting in instrument crowding. Instrument crowding is partially responsible for the challenges of suturing with the da Vinci Surgical Robot in the airway. The primary reason is the limited distal dexterity of the instruments, which lack the ability to roll, the key motion in passing a curved needle. Rahbar and colleagues [24] were able to suture two laryngeal clefts, albeit with the endosuture technique. Additionally, because of the robotic arm opposition, the procedure is performed with a wide angle between instruments resulting in a technically complex and awkward operation. Last, the $1.5 million initial cost and

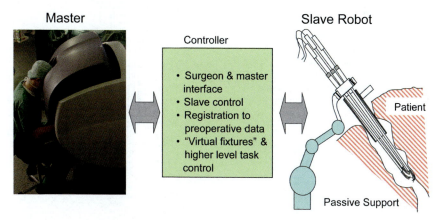

Fig. 3. Experimental design for laryngeal minimally invasive surgery contains a slave robot with two to three coaxial arms.

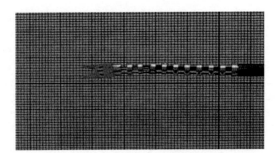

Fig. 4. Photo of 4-mm-diameter snakelike distal dexterity unit.

$100,000 annual service contract for the da Vinci Surgical Robot make it prohibitive for hospitals to acquire solely for airway procedures [12]. For the da Vinci system to be cost efficient, otolaryngologists likely will have to be at large hospitals that have purchased a robot for urologic, cardiothoracic, laparoscopic, and gynecologic applications [12].

Further advancements in robotic surgery are necessary to facilitate the entry of robotic surgery into the otolaryngologist's armamentarium. Future prototypes will incorporate instrument miniaturization, robot arms that function in the coaxial plane of the laryngoscope, integration of suction and powered instruments into the robots arms, and enhanced tool-tip dexterity. Our laboratory is developing a modular, scalable surgical robot to

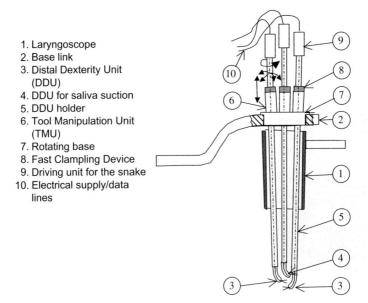

1. Laryngoscope
2. Base link
3. Distal Dexterity Unit
   (DDU)
4. DDU for saliva suction
5. DDU holder
6. Tool Manipulation Unit
   (TMU)
7. Rotating base
8. Fast Clampling Device
9. Driving unit for the snake
10. Electrical supply/data
    lines

Fig. 5. Conceptual design for coaxial three-armed slave robot with 4-mm snakelike distal dexterity units.

address the limitations of the current da Vinci Surgical Robot for applications in the airway (Fig. 3). A prototype has been designed with 4-mm-diameter snakelike instrument arms (Fig. 4). The snakelike arms are able to enter the laryngoscope in near parallel position and are designed with continuous backbones rather than pins or joints (Fig. 5). This central backbone design designed has the potential to deliver a variety of instruments including a laser, suction, drill, and other powered instruments. The arms are controlled by compact tool manipulation units at the proximal end well outside of the field of surgery. Enhanced tool-tip dexterity (distal dexterity) is provided with a flexible snakelike motion as compared with the articulating endowrist design of the da Vinci Robot. The increased distal flexibility improves the robot's ability to maneuver in the small operative space of the airway, enabling suturing and functional reconstruction of tissue (Fig. 6). The snakelike robot is specialized for minimally invasive surgery of the airway and is not modeled after the human arm. The small arm size and unique motion of robotic arms is designed to use less volume of motion to perform a surgical task. Each robotic arm has two snakelike units that may be

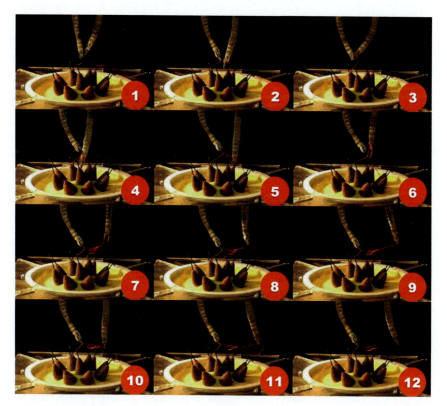

Fig. 6. Twelve-photo sequence demonstrating the progression of two distal dexterity units tying a knot with a suture.

compared with the curve of a finger. Each robotic arm has eight DoF with the proximal actuators capable of moving up and down, moving right and left, moving in and out, and roll. Furthermore, each of the two snakelike units within the arm is capable of yaw and pitch.

Application of robotics to laryngeal surgery will enhance surgical precision and open the door to other minimally invasive procedures not feasible with current instrumentation. This system would facilitate resection of small lesions, such as papillomas or carcinomas, and suture repair of surgical and traumatic defects. An efficient and accurate suturing method would improve the repair of laryngeal microflaps, glottic web flaps, and laryngeal clefts; secure cartilage grafts; and reposition vocal folds. Further utility would be seen in repair of tracheo-esophageal fistulas, endoscopic positioning of arytenoids, and medialization and lateralization procedures, and would refine endoscopic cricoid split procedures for airway expansion [27]. Outside of laryngology, a multi-armed robotic system would have utility in microvascular surgery, procedures at the base of the skull, sinus surgery, and single-port gastrointestinal and thoracic access surgery.

References

[1] Plinkert P, Lowenheim H. Trends and perspectives in minimally invasive surgery in otorhinolaryngology-head and neck surgery. Laryngoscope 1997;107:1483–9.
[2] Lynch RC. Suspension laryngoscopy and its accomplishments. Ann Otol Rhinol Laryngol 1915;24:429–78.
[3] von Leden H. Microlaryngoscopy: a historical vignette. J Voice 1988;1:341–6.
[4] Jako GJ. Laryngoscope for microscopic observation, surgery, and photography. The development of an instrument. Arch Otolaryngol 1970;91:196–9.
[5] Kleinsasser O. Microsurgery of the larynx. Arch Ohren Nasen Kehlkopfheilkd 1964;183: 428–33 [in German].
[6] Jako GJ. Laser surgery of the vocal cords. An experimental study with carbon dioxide lasers on dogs. Laryngoscope 1972;82:2204–16.
[7] Strong MS, Jako GJ. Laser surgery in the larynx. Early clinical experience with continuous CO2 laser. Ann Otol Rhinol Laryngol 1972;81:791–8.
[8] Myer CM 3rd, Willging JP, McMurray S, et al. Use of a laryngeal micro resector system. Laryngoscope 1999;109:1165–6.
[9] Patel N, Rowe M, Tunkel D. Treatment of recurrent respiratory papillomatosis in children with the microdebrider. Ann Otol Rhinol Laryngol 2003;112:7–10.
[10] Woo P, Casper J, Griffin B, et al. Endoscopic microsuture repair of vocal fold defects. J Voice 1995;9:332–9.
[11] Fleming DJ, McGuff S, Simpson CB. Comparison of microflap healing outcomes with traditional and microsuturing techniques: initial results in a canine model. Ann Otol Rhinol Laryngol 2001;110:707–12.
[12] Weinstein GS, O'Malley BW Jr, Snyder W, et al. Transoral robotic surgery: supraglottic partial laryngectomy. Ann Otol Rhinol Laryngol 2007;116:19–23.
[13] Chitwood WR Jr, Nifong LW, Chapman WH, et al. Robotic surgical training in an academic institution. Ann Surg 2001;234:475–84.
[14] Binder J, Brautigam R, Jonas D, et al. Robotic surgery in urology: fact or fantasy? BJU Int 2004;94:1183–7.

[15] Boehm DH, Arnold MB, Detter C, et al. Incorporating robotics into an open-heart program. Surg Clin North Am 2003;83:1369–80.

[16] Diodato MD Jr, Damiano RJ Jr. Robotic cardiac surgery: overview. Surg Clin North Am 2003;83:1351–67.

[17] Hockstein NG, Nolan JP, O'Malley BW Jr, et al. Robotic microlaryngeal surgery: a technical feasibility study using the daVinci surgical robot and an airway mannequin. Laryngoscope 2005;115:780–5.

[18] McLeod IK, Melder PC. Da Vinci robot-assisted excision of a vallecular cyst: a case report. Ear Nose Throat J 2005;84:170–2.

[19] Hockstein NG, Nolan JP, O'Malley BW Jr, et al. Robot-assisted pharyngeal and laryngeal microsurgery: results of robotic cadaver dissections. Laryngoscope 2005;115:1003–8.

[20] Hockstein NG, O'Malley BW Jr, Weinstein GS. Assessment of intraoperative safety in transoral robotic surgery. Laryngoscope 2006;116:165–8.

[21] O'Malley BW Jr, Weinstein GS, Hockstein NG. Transoral robotic surgery (TORS): glottic microsurgery in a canine model. J Voice 2006;20:263–8.

[22] O'Malley BW Jr, Weinstein GS, Snyder W, et al. Transoral robotic surgery (TORS) for base of tongue neoplasms. Laryngoscope 2006;116:1465–72.

[23] Weinstein GS, O'Malley BW Jr, Hockstein NG. Transoral robotic surgery: supraglottic laryngectomy in a canine model. Laryngoscope 2005;115:1315–9.

[24] Rahbar R, Ferrari LR, Borer JG, et al. Robotic surgery in the pediatric airway: application and safety. Arch Otolaryngol Head Neck Surg 2007;133:46–50.

[25] Mack MJ. Minimally invasive and robotic surgery. JAMA 2001;285:568–72.

[26] McLeod IK, Mair EA, Melder PC. Potential applications of the da Vinci minimally invasive surgical robotic system in otolaryngology. Ear Nose Throat J 2005;84:483–7.

[27] Inglis AF Jr, Perkins JA, Manning SC, et al. Endoscopic posterior cricoid split and rib grafting in 10 children. Laryngoscope 2003;113:2004–9.

ELSEVIER
SAUNDERS

Otolaryngol Clin N Am
41 (2008) 793–818

OTOLARYNGOLOGIC
CLINICS
OF NORTH AMERICA

Effects of Laryngeal Cancer on Voice and Swallowing

Heather M. Starmer, MA, CCC-SLP[a],
Donna C. Tippett, MPH, MA, CCC-SLP[a,b],
Kimberly T. Webster, MA, MS, CCC-SLP[a,*]

[a]*Department of Otolaryngology, Head and Neck Surgery, Johns Hopkins University,
601 N. Caroline Street, Room 6265, Baltimore, MD 21287, USA*
[b]*Department of Physical Medicine and Rehabilitation, Johns Hopkins University,
601 N. Caroline Street, Baltimore, MD 21287, USA*

Verbal communication relies on voice production in concert with other factors such as language, resonance, and articulation. Voice is generated when expiratory air passes through the approximated vocal folds, causing them to vibrate. The quality of sound produced depends on a number of factors including subglottic air pressure, degree of glottic closure, and the vibratory properties of the vocal folds. When discussing the voice, it is important to consider that for many people the voice is not just a tool for communication, but also an identifying feature that allows expression of personality.

Oral nutrition encompasses the natural but neuromuscularly complex acts of eating and swallowing. Both voluntary and involuntary actions are involved. Eating and swallowing are vital to life sustenance and also allow for a myriad of social interactions. Any difficulty in this area makes one appreciate the functions that most people take for granted.

Laryngeal cancer can have a dramatic impact on this delicately balanced system leading to disturbances of voice and swallowing. Increased mass of the vocal fold is predicted based on the presence of an invasive lesion. Other changes include irregularity of the vocal fold edge and/or reduced mobility both of which can lead to glottic incompetence [1]. These changes impact the vibratory characteristics of the vocal folds and often lead to marked dysphonia. Patients with laryngeal carcinoma frequently complain of hoarseness, reduced loudness, increased vocal effort, breathy voice, or painful voice

* Corresponding author. Johns Hopkins University, Baltimore, MD.
E-mail address: kwebste1@jhmi.edu (K.T. Webster).

0030-6665/08/$ - see front matter © 2008 Elsevier Inc. All rights reserved.
doi:10.1016/j.otc.2008.01.018

production. Larynx tumors can also cause odynophagia, obstruction, inco-ordination of swallowing musculature, increased oropharyngeal transit times and residue and sometimes aspiration [2]. Comprehensive evaluation by a speech-language pathologist before treatment is essential in document-ing pretreatment dysphonia and dysphagia, as well as allowing for patient education. Treatment for laryngeal cancer, including surgery, chemother-apy, radiotherapy and combined modality treatments can further compro-mise voice and swallowing function. In this article we discuss specific deficits that may be encountered as well as interventional strategies and evidence-based practice.

Surgical effects on voice and swallowing

Careful patient selection has led to improved oncologic control with la-ryngeal conservation procedures, making them increasingly attractive options for the treatment of laryngeal cancer [3]. In addition, many partial laryngectomy procedures are now done endoscopically [4]. A goal of conser-vation surgery is to minimize functional impact on voice production and swallowing.

The vocal folds are the vibratory sound source responsible for voice production. Any intervention that causes disruption in the vibratory charac-teristics of the vocal folds may result in dysphonia. Postoperative complica-tions such as disruption of laryngeal innervation, edema, and scar and granulation formation can complicate phonatory function. Generally speak-ing, voice therapy for surgical patients focuses on maximizing the natural qualities of the voice through phonation without excessive effort, improved air/muscle balance, and use of prosodic manipulations [5].

Surgical resection of the larynx can affect swallowing safety and effi-ciency. Careful evaluation with instrumental procedures and application of evidence-based swallowing intervention can yield positive functional outcomes. The following section describes common voice and swallowing difficulties following surgical procedures. Evidence-based research is cited where available.

Minimally invasive treatments

Laser excision and voice

Laser excision for early glottic carcinoma is one alternative to radiother-apy protocols. Cure rates are considered to be comparable for these modali-ties, ranging from 66% to 95% for patients undergoing radiotherapy and 76% to 96% for patients undergoing endoscopic laser excision [6]. Fre-quently, radiotherapy has been favored over laser excision due to reduced impact on the voice after treatment [7]. Extent of voice impact after resection is heavily dependent on the depth of the resection, with resections limited to the superficial layer of the lamina propria, Reinke's space, and the vocal ligament resulting in near normal voice production in most cases [8]. Deeper resections extending to the vocalis muscle can result in a significant increase in postoperative dysphonia [9]. Surgical interventions to address dysphonia after such deep resection may include microlaryngoscopic lipoinjection, medialization thyroplasty, and anterior commissure laryngoplasty [10]. Many patients will also require voice therapy following these procedures to maximize voice potential [10].

Common complaints regarding voice after laser excision include increased vocal effort, the need to take frequent breaths, and difficulty with pitch and loudness control [11]. Videostroboscopic assessment of these patients may reveal glottic incompetence, decreased mucosal wave, and vocal fold stiffness [8,9]. Despite complaints regarding voice after such procedures, patient-perceived voice handicap as measured by the Voice Handicap Index (VHI) is relatively low in contrast to other voice disorders. In a recent study by Brondbo and Benninger [12], patients after laser resection provided an overall score of 13 out of a possible 120 points on this measure indicating a low level of perceived limitation. Other authors report higher scores for dysphonia due to muscle tension dysphonia and unilateral paralysis [13].

Voice therapy for patients after laser excision will depend on their specific deficits and personal goals. In the immediate postoperative period, patients should be encouraged to comply with a period of total voice rest to facilitate healing. A recent study using a canine model is supportive of a rapid reestablishment of the basement membrane zone when a period of vocal rest is compared with a voice use condition [14]. Following the immediate postoperative period, a typical voice therapy protocol will include information regarding vocal hygiene and direct voice work. Use of voice therapy to improve both acoustic parameters and patient perceived handicap has been supported, although the specifics of the therapy protocol are not provided [15]. In this study an average improvement of 15 points on the VHI was reported after a course of voice therapy for a group of patients who had either a laser excision or radiotherapy. Despite improvement in functional outcomes, return to normal function was not observed.

Vocal hygiene recommendations are typically reviewed with patients during the education portion of treatment. Patients are advised to improve systemic and direct hydration; to avoid phonotraumatic behaviors such as yelling, shouting, and throat clearing; and to reduce laryngeal irritants such as acid reflux or smoke. Although vocal hygiene approaches have not been directly evaluated with this patient population, they have been validated in a number of studies involving teachers and professional voice users [16,17].

Voice intervention strategies are chosen based on the individual's deficits. Postoperatively, hyperfunction and hypofunction are possible. In general, treatment targets include improved glottic closure, reduced supraglottic tension, improved balance between airflow and muscular forces, and increased mobility of the laryngeal musculature. A number of techniques may be useful in this population including resonant voice therapy [18,19] and vocal function exercises [20]. In resonant voice therapy, the patient uses a barely adducted/abducted laryngeal posture to gain maximal vocal results with minimal impact stress and vocal effort. The vocal function exercises are a holistic approach to achieving air-muscle balance during phonation. Furthermore, these exercises directly modify vocal fold flexibility and can lead to improved vocal performance and endurance. Because of direct stretching accomplished with these exercises, they may contribute to improved flexibility of established scar tissue. When direct voice modification does not yield desired results in patients with hypofunction, use of small, personal voice amplifiers can be effective.

Laser excision and swallowing

The impact of endoscopic laser excision for laryngeal cancer on swallowing is similarly minimal. Preservation of laryngeal and pharyngeal movement and sensation with endoscopic procedures offers clear advantages over open procedures, radiotherapy, or chemoradiation. Size and location of tumor are important factors, however [21]. Reports of dysphagia after minimally invasive treatment for laryngeal cancer usually discuss T2-T4 glottic cancer, as treated T1 tumors have little to no effect on swallowing [22]. The need for a nasogastric (NG) feeding tube is usually temporary and duration of use correlates with size of tumor/extent of resection, but is generally less than 3 weeks [23]. In a study of 210 patients with laryngeal and hypopharyngeal cancer, Bernal-Sprekelsen and colleagues [23] report that 3.8% required a postoperative tracheotomy and 6.2% required a gastrostomy tube for dysphagia including aspiration. Postoperative radiation was related to more severe dysphagia in this and other studies [22]. Despite the trend toward worse functional outcomes on swallowing with adjuvant radiation and minimally invasive surgery, the study by Jepsen and colleagues [22] found important advantages with combined treatment modalities (surgery and radiation). In this group, no patients required tracheostomy or permanent gastrostomy and only 17% needed temporary nonoral feeding tubes. Comparable results have been noted across the age span [24].

In the cited articles, specific descriptions of dysphagia other than aspiration were not included. One study mentions that reduced pharyngeal constrictor motility and impaired pharyngeal and laryngeal sensation due to scarring and edema can account for dysphagia after endoscopic laser procedures for laryngeal cancer [25]. Specifics of dysphagia treatment are not common in the literature regarding patients undergoing minimally invasive procedures for larynx cancer. Medical/surgical management including autologous fat injection (AFI) has been described as helpful for dysphagia due to glottic insufficiency. Because of resorption of the fat, this may need to be repeated after several months, but in a study of 11 patients, 100%

were found to have improved swallowing 1 year after AFI [26]. Because of the risk of reduced sensation, instrumental procedures, such as videofluoroscopy (VFSS) or fiber-optic endoscopic evaluation of swallowing (FEES), are recommended to evaluate swallowing and plan appropriate treatment.

Partial laryngectomy

More extensive lesions of the larynx often require more aggressive surgical management such as vertical hemilaryngectomy, supraglottic laryngectomy, or supracricoid laryngectomy. The extent of functional deficits depends on the procedure completed. It is imperative that the patient meet with the speech pathologist before beginning treatment (surgical, nonsurgical, or combined modalities) to assess individual potential and motivation for rehabilitation. Particularly in the case of the supraglottic and supracricoid laryngectomy, the patient must be willing to commit to extensive rehabilitation to maximize potential for improvement. One cornerstone of such preoperative meetings should be emphasis of functional recovery versus return to normal function [27].

Vertical hemilaryngectomy and voice

In a standard vertical partial/hemilaryngectomy, one vertical half of the larynx is removed, transecting the thyroid cartilage and typically including one false vocal fold, one ventricle, and one true vocal fold. As a result, glottic incompetence and subsequent dysphonia are common. Preservation of the arytenoid, hyoid, and epiglottis is common [3,28]. Common findings following vertical hemilaryngectomy include incomplete glottic closure, assistance of the the supraglottic structures (ventricular folds, arytenoids) for abutement of the remaining fold, reduced maximum phonation time, high and more variable pitch, and restricted vocal intensity range. These patients often undergo additional procedures to improve glottic valving including medialization and reconstructive procedures. Despite elimination of glottic insufficiency, these patients often continue to report dysphonia secondary to alteration of their vibratory characteristics [11].

After vertical hemilaryngectomy, voice rehabilitation is geared toward compensation for deficits. In addition to surgical options to narrow the glottic gap, digital or external compression of the thyroid laminae can be used for improved glottic closure. A head turn to the affected side can also be useful. Other strategies can be implemented to reduce the functional impact of the dysphonia including use of amplification and environmental manipulation.

Vertical hemilaryngectomy and swallowing

Functional swallowing results after hemilaryngectomy are generally good relative to other partial laryngectomy procedures, with some initial difficulties in the early postoperative period. Most patients regain normal swallowing within 1 month of surgery [3,29,30]. With classical hemilaryng-ectomy, aspiration during the swallow is most prevalent, with some patients aspirating after the swallow or during and after [31].

Ideally, the operated side will abut against the intact side to achieve adequate laryngeal closure, allowing for safe swallowing. Some temporary postures or maneuvers may be necessary until this occurs consistently. If the primary problem is airway entrance closure, a chin tuck posture may reduce this risk by narrowing the potential opening. If both airway entrance and glottic closure are problematic, head turn to the damaged side with or without chin tuck may be helpful. The head rotation places extrinsic pressure on the thyroid cartilage, increasing adduction of the vocal fold to the reconstructed side of the larynx [32]. If postures alone are not sufficient in reducing aspiration, the supraglottic or super supraglottic swallow maneuvers can be attempted under fluoroscopy with or without the head postures to determine the best technique for maximal airway closure [29].

If surgery extends anteriorly to include the anterior commissure or part of the contralateral vocal fold or posteriorly to include the opposite arytenoid cartilage, patients may have more severe swallowing safety issues, requiring more intense and longer duration of swallowing therapy [28]. Jacob and colleagues [33] report on long-term functional outcomes after Laccourreye hemipharyngectomy-hemilaryngectomy for 22 patients. After a mean of 43 months, 14 reported normal eating and drinking while 6 could only eat soft foods, and 2 needed a permanent gastrostomy tube. If other deficits are identified during the evaluation, these should be addressed appropriately, as discussed in the following section of this article.

Supraglottic laryngectomy

Supraglottic laryngectomy and voice

Supraglottic carcinoma has been traditionally treated with open supraglottic or horizontal laryngectomy with good functional recovery of voice and swallowing in most patients [29,30]. Traditional open supraglottic laryngectomy (SGL) removes the epiglottis, both aryepiglottic folds, both false vocal folds, and one or both superior laryngeal nerves [34] and preserves both true vocal folds, both arytenoids, the base of tongue, and hyoid bone [3]. In the SGL, resection of the supraglottic larynx often results in alteration of the resonant characteristics of the voice. This results in a muffled voice that is difficult to project [27]. As a result, patients may be inclined to strain to produce a louder voice. Use of amplification may be helpful, particularly for patients who regularly have to project their voice.

Supraglottic laryngectomy and swallowing

With traditional open SGL, patients can begin eating some foods within 1 month of surgery but may take up to 3 months to return to a full oral diet

[29,35]. Extension of the SGL inferiorly or superiorly can prolong recovery, and dysphagia tends to be more severe, lasting 2 to 6 months and up to 2 years for some patients [29,36]. Higher T-stage of supraglottic tumors is also correlated with longer duration of feeding tubes [22]. Postoperative radiotherapy can further increase morbidity. Occasionally, safe swallowing is never achieved, requiring permanent means of nonoral feeding such as a gastrostomy tube or offering the patient conversion to total laryngectomy for chronic intractable aspiration/airway protection purposes [35]. Certainly, larger, more extensive, and more invasive resections, as well the addition of postoperative radiation therapy increase the possibility and severity of dysphagia symptoms. Subjective quality of life judgments after supraglottic laryngectomy show that dysphagia is directly related to size and extent of tumor [37].

Conversely, endoscopic laser resection of supraglottic tumors results in less dysphagia with more rapid return to normal swallowing, sometimes as rapidly as 2 to 7 days postoperatively [22,38]. One possible reason for improved outcomes in patients undergoing endoscopic SGL versus an open procedure is the preservation of the superior laryngeal nerve. Sasaki and colleagues [38] report an intact glottic closure reflex in six patients within 72 hours of surgery as demonstrated by testing with fiberoptic endoscopic evaluation of swallowing with sensory testing. In contrast, seven of eight patients post–open SGL had persistent loss of glottic closure reflex even up to 12 years.

With any of the SGL procedures, dysphagia is largely a function of airway protection problems [11,35]. Kreuzer and colleagues [31] performed videofluoroscopy on 120 laryngeal surgery patients and found aspiration to be common. In 61 partial laryngectomy patients who aspirated, 5 did so before the swallow, 32 during the swallow, 9 after the swallow, and 15 at more than one phase. The nature of aspiration was attributed to incomplete airway closure, sphincter dysfunction, or pharyngeal pooling. If the surgery is extended to include part or all of the hyoid bone, laryngeal elevation may be affected, contributing to reduced airway protection before or during the swallow. If the base of the tongue is involved, oropharyngeal transit and/or bolus control may be affected as well as bolus propulsion, resulting in residue after the swallow and/or risk of penetration and aspiration after the swallow [29,32].

Swallowing therapy can address each of the deficits listed above. As with any patient experiencing dysphagia, thorough clinical and instrumental examination, preferably videofluoroscopy, is performed to objectify deficits and plan treatment accordingly. Trial therapy techniques can be implemented and evaluated during the examination. These are necessary components for treatment planning with this population of patients [28,31,39].

Bolus control, lingual resistance, and other oral exercises can improve oral phase problems encountered [40,41]. Base of tongue exercises can improve retraction of the tongue base to the posterior pharyngeal wall. There are several voluntary maneuvers that achieve this, including effortful swallow, super-supraglottic swallow, Mendelsohn maneuver, and tongue-hold maneuver [42]. Specifically, the tongue-hold maneuver improves anterior movement of the posterior pharyngeal wall. Patients are instructed to protrude their tongue and hold it between their teeth while attempting to swallow. Additional therapy exercises used to improve tongue base retraction include yawn/sigh exercises, gargling, and simply instructing patients to retract their tongues as an exercise [43]. These are typically initiated during the postoperative evaluation and performed daily for 2 to 4 weeks. If no improvement is seen, continuing for another 4-week period is advisable [30].

The supraglottic swallow maneuver (SG) and the super-supraglottic swallow maneuver (SSG) are often indicated as both compensatory airway protection strategies and exercises [29,35]. Both teach the patient to maintain airway closure before and during the swallow. The SSG adds a voluntary Valsalva maneuver, increasing contact of the base of tongue to the arytenoids. The Mendelsohn maneuver is one way to improve laryngeal elevation and also increases and prolongs cricopharyngeal opening [44]. The Shaker exercise has been shown to improve upper esophageal opening associated with residue and aspiration after the swallow [45], although this can be difficult for patients having undergone surgery to the neck region. For persistent pharyngeal residue and aspiration after the swallow, which is not eliminated with above-described postures and maneuvers, side-lying posture may be effective. This posture eliminates the gravitational effect on pharyngeal residue, keeping it on one side of the pharynx [28,29,32]. Patients will usually need to implement a posture for 1 to 2 months and can return to normal eating without use of the posture after reassessment under videofluoroscopy to ensure that adequate improvement has occurred. Occasionally, postures may need to be used permanently [28].

Occasionally delayed pharyngeal swallow initiation occurs after SGL, further increasing the risk of aspiration, especially of thin liquids. This can be treated by having the patient compensate by volitionally holding liquids in the mouth briefly before swallowing. Some studies show reduced swallow delay using gustatory, mechanical, temperature (cold), and combined stimulation and temperature and texture variation of foods [29,46].

Medical/surgical procedures have a role in swallowing function with partial laryngectomy procedures. Both cricopharyngeal myotomy and pharyngeal plexus neurectomy at the time of partial laryngectomy have been shown to reduce dysphagia related to cricopharyngeal muscle spasm in supraglottic laryngectomy patients [47]. Electrical stimulation is emerging as a potential for dysphagia therapy. Although much more research needs to be completed, a promising intervention to date is the use of intramuscular hooked wire electrodes delivering paired stimulation to laryngeal elevation muscles. This shows the ability to induce laryngeal elevation and potentially improve patients with dysphagia due to reduced or delayed laryngeal elevation [48].

Supracricoid laryngectomy

The supracricoid laryngectomy (SCL) is based on the concept that the cricoarytenoid unit (arytenoid cartilage, cricoarytenoid joint, posterior and lateral cricoarytenoid muscles, and recurrent and superior laryngeal nerves) is the functional anatomic unit of the larynx [3]. This procedure includes the removal of the true and false vocal folds bilaterally, the bilateral paraglottic space, the entire thyroid cartilage, and at times the epiglottis and one arytenoid. This procedure, when used with stringent patient selection criteria, can lead to high local control (up to 98% at 5 years) while avoiding the need for a permanent tracheostoma [49]. This can result in significant improvement in overall quality of life in contrast to total laryngectomy (TL). Weinstein and colleagues [50] reported higher scores related to physical function, physical limitations, general health, vitality, social functioning, emotional limitations, and physical health summary as measured by the SF-36 for patients who underwent SCL versus TL.

Supracricoid laryngectomy and voice

Voice quality is significantly altered as a result of the supracricoid laryngectomy. Sound production depends on abutment of the remaining arytenoid against the epiglottis or tongue base [27]. Overall vocal quality was judged to be breathy-hoarse with a low fundamental frequency [51]. Despite the irregularity of voice after SCL, overall intelligibility is judged to be quite good (average score of 4 out of 5 possible by a blinded listener). Dworkin and colleagues [52] did not find any significant difference in the overall quality or intelligibility of voice produced after supracricoid laryngectomy in contrast to total laryngectomy with tracheoesophageal voice prosthesis (TEP). Of note, markedly lower neoglottal air forces were required for the SCL patients than the TL' patients (16 versus 31 cm H_2O), which may indicate lower vocal effort requirements in the SCL group. Vocal quality is expected to improve over time, although characteristics such as reduced frequency range, low fundamental frequency, and increased breathiness are expected to persist [53].

Voice therapy after supracricoid laryngectomy is again geared toward increasing function and compensation for deficits. Posterior tongue retraction can result in improved abutment of the arytenoid against the epiglottis or tongue base for increased voice [53]. As with other partial laryngectomy procedures, it is important to ensure that patients avoid strain and overcompensation [27], although with this population, some degree of overcompensation is necessary for functional outcomes.

Supracricoid laryngectomy and swallowing

Given that airway protection is compromised at the most inferior level of the larynx by the removal of the true and false vocal folds, therapy must focus on improved airway protection before and during the swallow [11]. Studies consistently show return to full oral diets and functional swallowing in 75% to 100% of patients [51,54,55]. Time from surgery to removal of feeding tubes has been cited as between 21 and 210 days [55]. Possible reasons for differences in time to recovery of functional swallowing include cricohyoidopexy (CHP) versus cricohyoidoepiglottopexy (CHEP), removal of one arytenoid cartilage in some patients and pre- or postoperative radiotherapy for some patients [55]. Others relate increased duration of nonoral feeding tubes to medical factors such as chronic obstructive pulmonary disease, diabetes mellitus, and increased time to tracheostomy tube removal [56]. Most studies report the importance of regular swallowing evaluation and therapy addressing a variety of oropharyngeal deficits. Characteristics of dysphagia include, but are not limited to, premature spillage, bolus retention, laryngeal penetration, aspiration, and ability to clear aspirated material by coughing [57]. Ruiz and Crevier-Buchman [58] describe a combination chin-down posture with base of tongue retraction in conjunction with a supraglottic swallow, which addresses many of these deficits. Other interventions as described in the previous and following sections of this article should be used as indicated by instrumental assessment.

Total laryngectomy

Removal of the entire larynx and separation of the upper and lower airways results in a significant alteration in the ability to verbally communicate. Voice production relies on an efferent air source, a vibrating body, and a resonant tract. In the case of total laryngectomy, the vibrating body is removed and there is alteration of the air source and resonant tract. The primary goal of postoperative voice therapy is to establish an alternative vibratory source. This can be accomplished using mechanical vibration, such as with an electrolarynx, or via vibration of the pharyngoesophageal segment (PES), such as with esophageal or tracheoesophageal speech. The key to successful functional outcomes and patient satisfaction, regardless of alaryngeal speech modality is patient education, before, during, and following treatment to develop realistic expectations.

Electrolaryngeal speech

Electrolaryngeal speech is accomplished by placing the electrolaryngeal device either on the neck, on the cheek, or intraorally. Once vibration is introduced, the patient uses the lips, tongue, teeth, and palate, as usual for articulation. Difficulties with electrolaryngeal speech can arise when the patient has difficulty obtaining adequate vibration due to placement or tissue properties, inadequate articulation, or suboptimal timing characteristics. Treatment for electrolaryngeal speech will address these difficulties using targeted speech drills and functional speech activities.

Esophageal speech

Esophageal speech requires active air injection into the esophagus through the pharyngoesophageal segment (PES). This can be accomplished through positive or negative pressure approaches. The patient then expels the air rapidly in an efferent manner causing vibration of the muscles and tissue of the cervical esophagus and hypopharynx. Postoperative therapy for esophageal speech includes instruction in air injection techniques, articulatory work, improvement of utterance length, and improved naturalness of speech. Esophageal speech, although once the mainstay of alaryngeal voice restoration, has less clinical popularity today because of lower levels of successful acquisition and poorer intelligibility ratings in contrast to tracheoesophageal speech [59,60]. In fact it is estimated that up to 75% of those attempting esophageal speech are unable to successfully acquire this modality [61].

Tracheoesophageal speech

The advent of the tracheoesophageal voice prosthesis (TEP) has revolutionized postoperative alaryngeal voice restoration [62]. At the time of the laryngectomy, or at a future date, a puncture is surgically created in the party wall between the trachea and esophagus. A one-way tracheoesophageal voice prosthesis is placed in the tract and when the stoma is occluded, air is shunted into the esophagus. The efferent air travels superiorly, causing the PES to vibrate. This sound source becomes the basis of alaryngeal communication in the TEP user. Recent reports of the successful long-term use of TE speech have revealed a range between 50% and 95% [63–65]. Voice quality ratings of fair-excellent have been reported in 88% of patients [63]. There are reports of improved outcomes for those undergoing primary puncture at the time of laryngectomy versus those undergoing a secondary puncture at a later date [66,67].

Difficulties with successful TEP use may be related to tonicity of the PES, difficulty with stomal occlusion, and prosthesis valve failure. Hypertonicity or spasm of the PES can lead to strained voice, effortful voice, and total inability to produce voice in up to 79% of those patients unable to achieve TE speech [68]. This problem is typically managed through medical/surgical approaches such as myotomy or injection of botulinum toxin [69–71]. Strictures within the esophagus can also impact voice production and are most often managed through dilatation. Issues with the PES can often be confirmed through videofluoroscopic evaluation.

Inadequate stomal occlusion because of stoma size, shape, or general neck topography can lead to air wasting and suboptimal airflow into the esophagus. In addition, excessive force applied by the patient can lead to narrowing of the vibrating region, leading to strained or absent voice. Both inadequate closure and excessive force are issues that can be addressed by the speech pathologist. Use of tracheostoma valves, housings, and intraluminal attachments can improve functional stomal occlusion, thereby facilitating TE speech. Creative management using devices such as the Barton Mayo button and the Provox Larytube and Laryclips can greatly enhance patient outcomes [72,73], particularly when paired with hands-free devices.

Voice prosthesis leakage is the most common maintenance issue with the TEP and can lead to reduction in long-term patient satisfaction [63]. Leakage can occur through the shaft of the prosthesis due to forces maintaining flap opening such as microbial colonization, valve deformities, or negative esophageal pressure during speech/swallowing. New prosthesis designs have targeted these issues through use of *Candida*-resistant materials, inset flap valves, and magnet closure systems [74–76]. Traditionally, use of Nystatin has been recommended to combat adhesion of *Candida* on the esophageal aspect of the prosthesis [77]; however, recent studies suggest that additional materials such as probiotics [78,79] and Amphoterican B lozenges may have additional benefits for reducing biofilm formation [80,81].

Leakage around the prosthesis, although less frequent in occurrence, can be a more difficult issue. Leakage around the prosthesis is often a result of excessive prosthesis length but can also be due to factors such as radiation effects, hypothyroidism, and recurrent cancer [82]. As a result, determination of the underlying cause of this leakage is critical. Remeasuring the length of the puncture tract and proper fitting of a new prosthesis can often eliminate leakage around the prosthesis. This is particularly the case for the first year after laryngectomy when edema and tissue thickness are gradually decreasing. Use of specialty prostheses with enlarged retention collars can also be used to prevent leakage around the prosthesis. Medical/surgical management for this problem can include injection of augmentation materials [83,84] or, in severe cases, closure of the tract with re-puncture at a subsequent date.

Total laryngectomy and swallowing

Although safety is not a typical concern after total laryngectomy, swallowing efficiency can be compromised by structural abnormalities and pharyngo-esophageal motility issues [29]. Videofluoroscopy is an effective method for detecting postsurgical structural abnormalities including early postoperative fistulas, strictures, and masses suspicious for recurrence [30], as well as pharyngoesophageal (PE) segment spasms and motility issues. Pharyngocutaneous fistula is an infrequent (17%–18% of patients) but real complication in this population that delays ability to resume oral diets [85,86]. There is some evidence that this is more common in patients having a salvage laryngectomy for recurrence after primary chemoradiation rather than a primary total laryngectomy [86] and in patients undergoing vertical versus "T" closure [85].

Other structural causes of dysphagia warrant intervention to directly improve swallowing. A pseudoepiglottis may form at the base of tongue, requiring laser excision if severe enough to cause backflow into the oro- or nasopharynx [29,85]. Stricture or narrowing of PES or esophagus can cause difficulty swallowing solids. Incidence of stricture after total laryngectomy may be as high as 39% [85] and has been cited as more common with more extensive surgeries such as laryngopharyngectomy with primary TEP [87]. Treatment with careful dilatation brings relief to many. Performing a cricopharyngeal (CP) myotomy at the time of total laryngectomy may avoid problems due to spasm at this site and retention of foods in the upper esophagus. Horowitz and Sasaki [88] measured peak pharyngeal pressures in TL patients with and without CP myotomy and found a significant difference, concluding that the procedure has the potential to minimize postoperative fistulization, eliminate dysphagia related to CP spasm, and improve acquisition of alaryngeal voice.

Without normal pharyngeal musculature, it is not surprising that many laryngectomees complain of increased effort swallowing and prolonged mealtimes. Direct swallowing therapy including base of tongue retraction exercises may improve dysphagia related to bolus transfer and manipulation difficulties [29]. A tongue-holding maneuver may improve anterior motion of the posterior pharyngeal wall [89], though this has not been studied in the TL population. Alternating liquids and solids and including moist or wet foods in all meals are helpful behavioral strategies.

Chemo- and radiation therapy effects on voice

Voice production and early glottic carcinoma

Although surgical approaches to laryngeal cancer have been fine-tuned to minimize functional impact on voice and swallowing, radiation therapy with and without chemotherapy remains an excellent option for management of early laryngeal cancer. In a review article by Kadish [90], local control rates for T1 and T2 laryngeal cancers treated with definitive radiation therapy were reported to be 80% to 93% for T1 and 65% to 78% for T2 disease. He further reports data for patients undergoing transoral laser excision to be from 88% to 93% for T1 lesions. With similar control rates, decisions regarding treatment modality depend heavily on functional impact of the different treatments. Simpson and colleagues [91] evaluated findings from a number of studies comparing voice quality after radiation versus laser excision. In three of the studies there was no difference in quality, and in the remainder there was a slight advantage for the patients who underwent radiation therapy.

Voice characteristics following organ preservation

Despite the favorable results obtained with radiation treatment, voice deficits can still be observed. It is, of course, important to consider that most patients will have experienced pretreatment dysphonia, which may be greater than what remains following treatment [92]. Forty-four percent of patients in a recent study by vanGogh and colleagues [15,93] suffered from voice impairment after radiotherapy based on responses to a screening questionnaire. This voice disturbance may be a result of radiation-induced tissue fibrosis, mucositis of soft tissues, atrophic changes, and mucosal changes due to xerostomia. Increased voice disturbance, decreased quality of life, and irregularity in stroboscopic evaluations have recently been linked to patients with xerostomia [94]. This study revealed significant changes in patients who received wide-field radiation therapy including the salivary glands but no significant change in patients who had narrow-field radiation for small glottic tumors. This study supports the notion that changes in hydration following radiation treatment to the lymphatic system can have marked impact on vocal function. In patients undergoing radiation therapy, stroboscopic evaluation may reveal reduced amplitude of vocal fold vibration, reduced mucosal wave, irregular phase symmetry, irregular glottic closure, and supraglottic compensation [95]. These stroboscopic findings are consistent with acoustic parameters such as reduced pitch range, reduced loudness, and reduced phrase length [7,92]. Furthermore, significant patient-reported handicaps have been measured using the VHI [15,96,97].

Voice therapy following organ preservation

Voice therapy can be implemented following radiation therapy to improve vocal quality, decrease patient-perceived vocal effort, and reduce voice-related handicap. A recent efficacy study by vanGogh and colleagues [15] found improvement in VHI scores and acoustic parameters after completion of voice therapy. Voice therapy in this population is designed to meet the needs of the patients and their specific deficits, which may be the result of tissue fibrosis, vocal fold atrophy, supraglottic compensation, and mucosal changes due to xerostomia. Techniques may target airflow and breath support, vocal fold pliability through pitch modulation, reduction in muscular tension, and manipulation of resonance. Resonant voice techniques including Lessac Madsen Resonant Voice Therapy [98] and Twang therapy [99] may be particularly useful in this population, as are vocal function exercises [20,100] and circumlaryngeal massage [101,102].

A key component of voice therapy after radiation is addressing hydration because of the strong link between xerostomia and voice disturbance. There is evidence to support use of Pilocarpines to address xerostomia following radiation [103,104]. Other treatments that have been linked to reduction of xerostomia effects include BioXtra mouth care products [105]; saliva substitutes containing hydroxyethyl-, hydroxypropyl-, or carboxymethylcellulose [106]; cevimeline [107]; and chewing gum with noncariogenic sweeteners [108]. Acupuncture has also been used successfully to improve xerostomia [109,110]. Behavioral techniques that may reduce patient complaints of xerostomia include increased water intake, increasing environmental humidification, steam inhalation, sucking on candy, elimination of dehydrating agents such as alcohol and caffeine, and use of saliva substitutes; however, these techniques have not been studied in regard to actual impact on xerostomia or voice production in irradiated patients. Improving hydration may result in improved vocal quality, reduced phonation threshold pressure, and reduced patient perception of vocal effort [111].

Voice production and late glottic carcinoma

Recently, cure rates are reported to be comparable for patients with advanced laryngeal cancer completing radiotherapy/chemotherapy as for patients undergoing total laryngectomy with postoperative radiation [112,113]. Furthermore, advances in delivery of radiotherapy including IMRT have led to theoretic reduction in functional impact following intervention, although studies have not yet been completed to confirm this. Despite these favorable findings, there remains evidence that radiologic and chemotherapeutic agents may have significant impact on voice production. These deficits have been attributed to radiation-induced fibrosis of the larynx and atrophy of the vocal folds as a result of radiation [114]. These postradiation changes can lead to voice complaints including vocal fatigue, decreased pitch range, reduced singing ability, decreased loudness, and decreased vocal clarity [11].

In 1999, Orlikoff and colleagues [115] used acoustic analysis, aerodynamic assessement, glottography, and videostroboscopy to evaluate posttreatment voice and laryngeal function. This study revealed significant abnormalities following treatment. A retrospective review by Meleca and colleagues [114] looked at functional outcomes for patients with stage III and IV laryngeal cancer after radiation or combined chemo/radiation treatment Their findings revealed increased acoustic instability, glottic incompetence; moderately deviant perceptual output in prosody, vocal quality, and intelligibility; increased pooling of thick saliva; reduced vocal fold mobility and vibration; and increased mobilization of the ventricular folds, but only mild voice handicap. Furthermore, they found that elapsed time posttreatment had a positive impact on patient perception of handicap, but not on actual measurements of voice and laryngeal function. Their findings regarding posttreatment voice changes are consistent with earlier studies [115]. Although greater functional impact may be expected in patients with advanced cancers, treatment strategies will not vary significantly from those described in the previous section.

Chemo- and radiation therapy effects on swallowing

Functional outcomes

Dysphagia and consequent diet modifications and weight loss are well-documented in those receiving nonsurgical treatment, although improved functional status and quality of life occur over time [116–119]. Individuals receiving nonsurgical treatments report that eating returns to normal to near-normal levels [114] and that quality of life approximates pretreatment levels several months after treatment [120]. Gillespie and colleagues [121] found no significant differences in emotional and functional status for surgery/radiation and chemoradiation groups with laryngeal/hypopharyngeal cancer sites.

Instrumental assessment

Dysphagia characteristics specific to those receiving nonsurgical treatment for laryngeal cancer are available. Carrara-de Angelis and colleagues [122] described reduced bolus formation, reduced bolus propulsion, oral stasis, pharyngeal stasis, laryngeal penetration, and aspiration on videofluoroscopic swallowing studies (VFSS) of 14 individuals who were treated with chemoradiation for advanced squamous cell carcinoma of the larynx or hypopharynx. At follow-up (mean = 20 months), seven patients had normal swallowing and only one patient was still using a gastrostomy feeding tube. Logemann and colleagues [123] reported that 28% of the patients with laryngeal cancer had gastrostomy tubes and 14% were aspirating before chemoradiation. Three months after treatment, the laryngeal cancer group had the highest frequency of reduced base of tongue retraction, reduced anterior-posterior tongue movement, delayed pharyngeal swallow, reduced laryngeal elevation, and reduced cricopharyngeal opening compared with nasopharyngeal, oropharyngeal, and hypopharyngeal cancer and unknown location groups. Half of these patients had their gastrostomy feeding tubes posttreatment and 7% continued to aspirate. Fiber-optic endoscopic swallowing study findings include premature spillage into the vallecula, vallecular and post cricoid retention, laryngeal penetration, and aspiration in individuals who received chemoradiation for advanced laryngeal carcinoma [124].

In several studies, patients with laryngeal cancer are included; however, site-specific data are not reported. Common decompensations include laryngeal penetration and aspiration, reduced posterior tongue base retraction, reduced laryngeal elevation, and need for multiple swallows to clear pharyngeal residue [125–127]. In other studies, dysphagia is reported in individuals treated nonsurgically for laryngeal cancer, but not specifically characterized [128,129]. Pretreatment data reveal disruption of normal swallowing in those with head and neck tumors [130,131].

Iatrogenic complications

Iatrogenic complications associated with nonsurgical treatment can exacerbate dysphagia. Mucositis, a primary complication of chemotherapy, can persist for weeks following completion of treatment, causing oral and pharyngeal tenderness and pain as well as sensitivity to temperature and spicy or acidic foods [132]. Complications associated with radiotherapy can be acute or late onset and include mucositis, candidiasis, dysgeusia, dental caries, osteoradionecrosis, soft tissue necrosis, and xerostomia [133].

IMRT provides highly conformal dose distribution around tumor targets and potentially spares mucosa and salivary glands [134,135]. Medications may also be used to either protect salivary glands or to improve salivary flow [136,137]. Dentifrices can be used to ameliorate dry mouth [138]. Oral intake is advocated during and after treatment to avoid stricture formation [125]. Range of movement exercises, stacked tongue blades, and specialized medical devices are used to treat trismus [139].

Treatment

Evidence-based practice begins with asking a clinical question and then investigating sources of support for answers. Clinical judgment, patient values, and research evidence must be critically appraised and integrated [140,141]. Speech-language pathologists can look forward to the results of two randomized clinical trials that include individuals with head/neck cancer to aid in rendering treatment decisions [142]. In the interim, supportive, rigorous evidenced-based client-specific research is difficult to identify and so the question "*Does* this treatment work?" remains unanswered. Nevertheless, clinicians can combine several lower-level studies of sufficiently good design, expert consensus, and clinical knowledge of anatomy and physiology to address the question "*Should* this treatment work?" [143]. For example, Kotz and colleagues [125] recommended effortful swallow, tongue base retraction exercises, falsetto voice exercises, suprasuperglottic swallow, and Mendelsohn maneuver based on the swallowing abnormalities observed in their patients with advanced head and neck cancer.

Exercises

Historically, the contribution of exercises in dysphagia treatment has been questioned. Perlman and colleagues [144] showed that employment of aerodynamic musculature is strongest during swallowing when compared with other aerodigestive functions, supporting the perspective that one should treat at a task level (ie, therapeutic swallowing, maneuvers that incorporate swallowing), consistent with the exercise physiology principle of specificity [145,146]. In some circumstances, treatment at a task level may be inappropriate, as in the case of the individual with recurrent pneumonia, flagrant aspiration, and risk factors known to predispose one to aspiration pneumonia [147]. An alternative is to identify and treat underlying impairments according to the concept of transference, which is the rationale for using a nonspecific task to improve a specifically defined behavior [148].

There is a resurgence of interest in oral motor exercises, particularly in the head and neck cancer population. Kulbersh and colleagues [149] found that patients undergoing radiation or chemoradiation protocols who performed pretreatment swallowing exercises showed significant improvement on self-reports of global, emotional and physical function compared with those who received posttreatment therapy. Their pretreatment protocol included the Mendelsohn maneuver, Shaker exercise, tongue hold, tongue resistance, and falsetto phonation.

Many questions persist regarding treatment of underlying deficits pertaining to isolation of individual muscles versus muscle groups, recovery time, and prescription of exercise dosage and frequency. Sound clinical practice should include identification of the therapy target (ie, strength, endurance, power), the rationale for treatment, baseline assessment, and documentation of changes in swallowing, weight, and quality of life [145].

Compensatory strategies

Based on instrumental swallowing study findings, relevant compensatory strategies are effortful swallow, Mendelsohn maneuver, and behavioral strategies, such as alternating solid and liquid consistencies. Chin tuck may be appropriate when oral control is compromised. Logemann and colleagues [150] found that fewer swallowing decompensations were observed when head and neck cancer patients who underwent radiotherapy and chemotherapy used the super-supraglottic swallow.

Diet modifications

Significant diet modifications should be preceded by compensatory strategies and postures. Softer, moister foods can facilitate swallowing in those with xerostomia and odynophagia. Use of thickened liquids should be considered carefully because of the implications for hydration/nutrition, quality of life, cost, noncompliance, and product variability [151,152].

Other considerations

The treatment of dysphagia is evolving to encompass a more holistic view of patients' health. Ashford and Mills [153] caution that an elevated neutrophil count and aspiration are optimal conditions for the development of pneumonia, and advise that laboratory values can be used to assist in decision making regarding methods of nutrition. Poor oral hygiene is a known risk factor for the development of pneumonia. Daily and professional oral hygiene appears to be an important component of illness prevention [154,155].

In conclusion, working with patients with laryngeal cancer on voice and swallowing rehabilitation is a challenging, but rewarding, experience. While assessment and treatment are always individualized, certain protocols are suggested, including pretreatment education and evaluation with a speech-language pathologist, careful instrumental assessment, and treatment plans that use evidence-based research. Coordination of treatment with other members of the head and neck cancer team can streamline appointments and reinforce team goals. The goal of voice and swallowing intervention is to restore functional outcomes of communication and oral nutrition, keeping patient and family goals paramount.

References

[1] Orlikoff RF, Kraus DH. Dysphonia following nonsurgical management of advanced laryngeal carcinoma. Am J Speech Lang Pathol 1996;5(3):47–52.

[2] Stenson KM, MacCracken E, List M, et al. Swallowing function in patients with head and neck cancer prior to treatment. Arch Otolaryngol Head Neck Surg 2000;126:371–7.

[3] Tufano R. Organ preservation for laryngeal cancer. Otolaryngol Clin North Am 2002; 35(5):1067–80.

[4] Moreau PR. Treatment of laryngeal carcinomas by laser endoscopic microsurgery. Laryngoscope 2000;110(6):1000–6.

[5] Doyle PC. Voice refinement following conservation surgery for cancer of the larynx: a conceptual framework for treatment intervention. Am J Speech Lang Pathol 1997;6:27–35.

[6] Peeters A, van Gogh C, Goor K, et al. Health status and voice outcome after treatment for T1a glottic carcinoma. Eur Arch Otorhinolaryngol 2004;261:534–40.

[7] Krengli M, Policarpo M, Manfredda I, et al. Voice quality after treatment for T1a glottic carcinoma. Acta Oncol 2004;43(3):284–9.

[8] Ledda GP, Grover N, Pundir V, et al. Functional outcomes after CO2 laser treatment of early glottic carcinoma. Laryngoscope 2006;116(6):1007–11.

[9] Zeitels SM. Phonomicrosurgical treatment of early glottic cancer and carcinoma in situ. Am J Surg 1996;172(6):704–9.

[10] Zeitels SM. Optimizing voice after endoscopic partial laryngectomy. Otolaryngol Clin North Am 2004;37(3):627–36.

[11] Samlan R, Webster K. Swallowing and speech therapy after definitive treatment for laryngeal cancer. Otolaryngol Clin North Am 2002;35:1115–33.

[12] Brondbo K, Benninger M. Laser resection of T1a glottic carcinomas: results and postoperative voice quality. Acta Otolaryngol 2004;124:976–9.

[13] Murry T, Rosen C. Outcome measurements and quality of life in voice disorders. Otolaryngol Clin North Am 2000;33:905–16.

[14] Cho SH, Kim HT, Lee IJ, et al. Influence of phonation on basement membrane zone recovery after phonomicrosurgery: a canine model. Ann Otol Rhinol Laryngol 2000; 109:658–66.

[15] Van Gogh CD, Verdonck-de Leeuw IM, Boon-Kamma BA, et al. The efficacy of voice therapy in patients after treatment for early glottic carcinoma. Cancer 2006;106(1): 95–105.

[16] Yiu EM, Chan RM. Effect of hydration and vocal rest on the vocal fatigue in amateur karaoke singers. J Voice 2003;17:216–27.

[17] Pederson M, Beranova A, Moller S. Dysphonia: medical treatment and a medical voice hygiene advice approach: a prospective randomized pilot study. Eur Arch Otorhinolaryngol 2004;261:312–5.

[18] Verdolini K. Resonant voice therapy. In: Stemple J, editor. Voice therapy: clinical studies. 2nd edition. San Diego (CA): Singular Publishing; 2000. p. 46–62, 85–96.

[19] Chen SH, Hsiao TY, Hsiao LC, et al. Outcome of resonant voice therapy for female teachers with voice disorders: perceptual, physiological, acoustic, aerodynamic, and functional measurements. J Voice 2006;21:415–25.

[20] Stemple JC. A holistic approach to voice therapy. Semin Speech Lang 2005;26(2):131–7.

[21] Hoffman HT, Buatti J. Update on the endoscopic management of laryngeal cancer. Curr Opin Otolaryngol Head Neck Surg 2004;12:525–31.

[22] Jepsen MC, Gurushanthaiah D, Roy N, et al. Voice, speech, and swallowing outcomes in laser-treated laryngeal cancer. Laryngoscope 2003;113:923–8.

[23] Bernal-Sprekelsen M, Vilaseca-Gonzalez I, Blanch-Alejandro JL. Predictive values for aspiration after endoscopic laser resections of malignant tumors of the hypopharynx and larynx. Head Neck 2004;26(2):103–10.

[24] Sesterhenn AM, Dunne AA, Werner JA. Complications after CO2 laser surgery of laryngeal cancer in the elderly. Acta Otolaryngol 2006;126:530–5.

[25] Brehmer D, Laubert A. Diagnosis of postoperative dysphagia and aspiration. Fiberoptic-endoscopic controlled methylene blue drinking. HNO 1999;47(5):479–84.

[26] Guven M, Suoglu Y, Kyak E, et al. Autologous fat injection for voice and swallow improvement after cordectomy. ORL J Otorhinolaryngol Relat Spec 2006;68:164–9.

[27] Sparano A, Ruiz C, Weinstein GS. Voice rehabilitation after external partial laryngeal surgery. Otolaryngol Clin North Am 2004;37(3):637–53.

[28] Logemann JA. Swallowing disorders after treatment for laryngeal cancer. In: Logemann JA, editor. Evaluation and treatment of swallowing disorders. 2nd edition. Austin (TX): PRO-ED; 1998.

[29] Lazarus CL. Management of swallowing disorders in head and neck cancer patients: optimal patterns of care. Semin Speech Lang 2000;21(4):293–309.

[30] Rademaker AW, Logemann JA, Pauloski BR, et al. Recovery of postoperative swallowing in patients undergoing partial laryngectomy. Head Neck 1993;15(4):325–34.

[31] Kreuzer SH, Schima W, Schober E, et al. Complications after laryngeal surgery: video-fluoroscopic evaluation of 120 patients. Clin Radiol 2000;55(10):775–81.

[32] Logemann JA, Rademaker AW, Pauloski LA, et al. Effects of postural change on aspiration in head and neck surgical patients. Otolaryngol Head Neck Surg 1994;10: 222–7.

[33] Jacob R, Zorowka P, Welkoborsky HJ, et al. Long-term functional outcome of Laccourreye hemipharyngectomy-hemilaryngectomy with reference to oncologic outcome. Laryngorhinootologie 1998;77(2):93–9.

[34] Weaver AW, Fleming SM. Partial laryngectomy: analysis of associated swallowing disorders. Am J Surg 1978;136(4):486–9.

[35] Logemann JA, Gibbons P, Rademaker AW, et al. Mechanisms of recovery of swallow after supraglottic laryngectomy. J Speech Hear Res 1994;37:965–74.

[36] Wasserman T, Murry T, Johnson JT, et al. Management of swallowing in supraglottic and extended supraglottic laryngectomy patients. Head Neck 2001;23:1043–8.

[37] Strek P, Hydzik-Sobocintska K, Skladzien J, et al. Self-assessment of the effect of dysphagia on the quality of life in patients after partial laryngectomy for cancer initially located in the supraglottic area. Pol Merkur Lekarski 2005;19(111):362–4.

[38] Sasaki CT, Leder SB, Acton LM, et al. Comparison of the glottic closure reflex in traditional "open" versus endoscopic laser supraglottic laryngectomy. Ann Otol Rhinol Laryngol 2006;115(2):93–6.

[39] Logemann JA. The dysphagia diagnostic procedure as a treatment efficacy trial. Clin Commun Disord 1993;3(4):1–10.

[40] Sonies BC. Remediation challenges in treating dysphagia post head/neck cancer. A problem-oriented approach. Clin Commun Disord 1993;3(4):21–6.

[41] Robbins J, Gangnon RE, Theis SM, et al. The effects of lingual exercise on swallowing in older adults. J Am Geriatr Soc 2005;53(9):1483–9.

[42] Lazarus C, Logemann JA, Song CW, et al. Effects of voluntary maneuvers on tongue base function for swallowing. Folia Phoniatr Logop 2002;54(4):171–6.

[43] Veis S, Logemann JA, Colangelo L. Effects of three techniques on maximum posterior movement of the tongue base. Dysphagia 2000;15(3):142–5.

[44] Lazarus C, Logemann JA, Gibbons P. Effects of maneuvers on swallowing function in a dysphagiac oral cancer patient. Head and Neck 1993;15:419–24.

[45] Shaker R, Easterling C, Kern M, et al. Rehabilitation of swallowing by exercise in tube-fed patients with pharyngeal dysphagia secondary to abnormal UES opening. Gastroenterology 2002;122(5):1314–21.

[46] Sciortino K, Liss JM, Case JL, et al. Effects of mechanical, cold, gustatory, and combined stimulation to the human anterior faucial pillars. Dysphagia 2003;18(1):16–26.

[47] Ceylan A, Koybasioglu A, Asal K, et al. The effects of pharyngeal neurectomy and crico-pharyngeal myotomy on postoperative deglutition in patients undergoing horizontal supra-glottic laryngectomy. Kulak Burun Bogaz Ihtis Derg 2003;11(6):170–4.

[48] Burnett TA, Mann EA, Cornell SA, et al. Laryngeal elevation achieved by neuromuscular stimulation at rest. J Appl Physiol 2003;94(1):128–34.

[49] Laccourreye O, Muscatello L, Laccourreye L, et al. Supracricoid partial laryngectomy with cricohyoidepiglottopexy for "early" glottic carcinoma classified as T1-T2N0 invading the anterior commissure. Am J Otolaryngol 1997;18(6):385–90.

[50] Weinstein GS, El-Sawy MM, Ruiz C, et al. Laryngeal preservation with supracricoid partial laryngectomy results in improved quality of life when compared with total laryngectomy. Laryngoscope 2001;111(2):191–9.

[51] Zacharek MA, Pasha R, Meleca RJ, et al. Functional outcomes after supracricoid laryngectomy. Laryngoscope 2001;111(9):1558–64.

[52] Dworken JP, Meleca RJ, Zacharek MA, et al. Voice and deglutition functions after the supracricoid and total laryngectomy procedures for advanced stage laryngeal carcinoma. Otolaryngol Head Neck Surg 2003;129(4):311–20.

[53] Crevier-Buchman L, Laccourreye O, Weinstein GS, et al. Evolution of speech and voice following supracricoid partial laryngectomy. J Laryngol Otol 1995;109:410–3.

[54] Lallemant JG, Bonnin P, el-Sioufi I, et al. Cricohyoepiglottopexy: long-term results in 55 patients. J Laryngol Otol 1999;113(6):532–7.

[55] Farrag TY, Koch WM, Cummings CW, et al. Supracricoid laryngectomy outcomes: the Johns Hopkins experience. Laryngoscope 2007;117:129–32.

[56] Marioni G, Marchese-Ragona R, Ottaviano G, et al. Supracricoid laryngectomy: is it time to define guidelines to evaluate functional results? A review. Am J Otolaryngol 2004;25: 98–104.

[57] Schindler A, Favero E, Nudo S, et al. Long-term voice and swallowing modifications after supracricoid laryngectomy: objective, subjective and self-assessment data. Am J Otolaryngol 2006;27:378–83.

[58] Ruiz C, Crevier-Buchman L. Swallowing rehabilitation following organ preservation surgery. In: Weinstein GS, Laccourreye O, Brasnu D, et al, editors. Organ preservation surgery for laryngeal cancer. San Diego (CA): Singular Publishing Group; 2000. p. 165–70.

[59] Doyle PC, Danhauer JL, Reed CG. Listeners perceptions of consonants produced by esophageal and tracheoesophageal talkers. J Speech Hear Dis 1988;53(4):400–7.

[60] Hyman M. An experimental study of artificial larynx and esophageal speech. J Speech Hear Dis 1955;20:291–9.

[61] Gates GA, Ryan W, Cooper JC, et al. Current status of laryngectomy rehabilitation: results of therapy. Am J Otolaryngol 1982;3:1–7.

[62] Singer MI, Blom ED. An endoscopic technique for restoration of voice after laryngectomy. Ann Otol Rhinol Laryngol 1980;89(6):529–33.

[63] Op de Coul BM, Hilgers FJ, Balm AJ, et al. A decade of postlaryngectomy vocal rehabilitation in 318 patients: a single institution's experience with consistent application of provox indwelling voice prostheses. Arch Otolaryngol Head Neck Surg 2000;126(11): 1320–8.

[64] Ferrer Ramirez MJ, Guallart Domenech F, Brotons Durban S, et al. Surgical voice restoration after total laryngectomy: long-term results. Eur Arch Otorhinolaryngol 2001;258(9):463–6.

[65] Mendenhall WM, Morris CG, Stringer SP, et al. Voice rehabilitation after total laryngectomy and postoperative radiation therapy. J Clin Oncol 2002;20(10):2500–5.

[66] Cheng E, Ho Mm, Ganz C, et al. Outcomes of primary and secondary tracheoesophageal puncture: a 16 year retrospective analysis. Ear Nose Throat J 2006;85(4):264–7.

[67] Chone CT, Gripp FM, Spina AL, et al. Primary versus secondary tracheoesophageal puncture for speech rehabilitation in total laryngectomy: long-term results with indwelling voice prosthesis. Otolaryngol Head Neck Surg 2005;133(1):89–93.

[68] Baugh RF, Lewin JS, Baker SR. Vocal rehabilitation of tracheoesophageal speech failures. Head Neck 1990;12(1):69–73.

[69] Op de Coul BM, van den Hoogen FJ, van As CJ, et al. Evaluation of the effects of primary myotomy in total laryngectomy on the neoglottis with the use of quantitative videofluoroscopy. Arch Otolaryngol Head Neck Surg 2003;129(9):1000–5.

[70] Hamaker RC, Blom ED. Botulinum neurotoxin for pharyngeal constrictor muscle spasm in tracheoesophageal voice restoration. Laryngoscope 2003;113(9):1479–82.

[71] Zormeier MM, Meleca RJ, Simpson ML, et al. Botulinum toxin injection to improve tracheoesophageal speech after total laryngectomy. Otolaryngol Head Neck Surg 1999; 120(3):314–9.

[72] Lewin JS. Nonsurgical management of the stoma to maximize tracheoesophageal speech. Otolaryngol Clin North Am 2004;37(3):585–96.

[73] Hilgers FJ, Ackerstaff A. Development and evaluation of a novel tracheostoma button and fixation system (Provox Larybutton and Laryclip adhesive) to facilitate hands-free tracheoesophageal speech. Acta Oto-Laryngol 2006;126(11):1218–24.

[74] Kress P, Schafer P, Schwerdtfeger FP. Clinical use of a voice prosthesis with a flap valve containing silver oxide (Blom Singer Advantage), biofilm formation, in-situ lifetime and indication. Laryngorhinootologie 2006;85(12):893–6.

[75] Leder SB, Acton LM, Kmiecik J, et al. Voice restoration with the Advantage tracheoesophageal voice prosthesis. Otolaryngol Head Neck Surg 2005;133:681–4.

[76] Hilgers FJ, Ackerstaff AH, Balm AJ, et al. A new problem-solving indwelling voice prosthesis, eliminating the need for frequent candida and "underpressure" related replacements: Provox ActiValve. Acta Otolaryngol 2003;123(8):972–9.

[77] Blom ED, Hamaker RC. Tracheoesophageal voice restoration following total laryngectomy. In: Meyers EN, Suen J, editors. Cancer of the head and neck. Philadelphia: W.B. Saunders; 1996. p. 839–52.

[78] Rodrigues L, van der Mei HC, Teixeira J, et al. Influence of biosurfactants from probiotic bacteria on formation of biofilms on voice prostheses. Appl Environ Microbiol 2004;70(7): 4408–10.

[79] Schwandt LQ, Van Weissenbruch R, Stokroos I, et al. Prevention of biofilm formation by dairy products and N-acetylcysteine on voice prostheses in an artificial throat. Acta Otolaryngol 2004;124(6):726–31.

[80] Paniagua GL, Monroy E, Negrete E, et al. Susceptibility to 5-fluorocytosine, miconazole, and amphotericin B of Candida albicans strains isolated from the throat of non-AIDS patients. Rev Latinoam Microbiol 2002;44(2):65–8.

[81] Aperis G, Myriounis N, Spanakis EK, et al. Developments in the treatment of candidiasis: more choices and new challenges. Expert Opin Investig Drugs 2006;15(11):1319–36.

[82] Bunting GM. Voice following laryngeal cancer surgery: troubleshooting common problems after tracheoesophageal voice restoration. Otolaryngol Clin North Am 2004;37: 597–612.

[83] Lorincz BB, Lichtenberger G, Bihari A, et al. Therapy of periprosthetical leakage with tissue augmentation using Bioplastique around the implanted voice prosthesis. Laryngology 2005;262:32–4.

[84] Seshamani M, Ruiz C, Schwartz Kasper, et al. Cymetra injections to treat leakage around a tracheoesophageal puncture. ORL J Otorhinolaryngol Relat Spec 2006;68(3):146–8.

[85] Davis RK, Vincent ME, Shapshay SM, et al. The anatomy and complications of "T" versus vertical closure of the hypopharynx after laryngectomy. Laryngoscope 1982;92:16–20.

[86] Ganly I, Patel S, Matsuo J, et al. Postoperative complications of salvage total laryngectomy. Cancer 2005;103(10):2073–81.

[87] Nyquist GG, Hier MP, Dionisopoulos T, et al. Stricture associated with primary tracheoesophageal puncture after pharyngolaryngectomy and free jejunal interposition. Head Neck 2006;28(3):205–9.

[88] Horowitz JB, Sasaki CT. Effect of cricopharyneus myotomy on postlaryngectomy pharyngeal contraction pressures. Laryngoscope 1993;103(2):138–40.

[89] Fujiu M. Effect of a tongue-holding maneuver on posterior pharyngeal wall movement during deglutition. Am J Speech Lang Pathol 1996;5(1):23–30.

[90] Kadish S. Can I treat this small larynx lesion with radiation alone? Update on the radiation management of early (T1 and T2) glottic cancer. Otolaryngol Clin North Am 2005;38(1):1–9.

[91] Simpson CB, Postma GN, Stone RE. Speech outcomes after laryngeal cancer management. Otolaryngol Clin N Amer 1997;30(2):189–205.

[92] Verdonck-de Leeuw IM, Hilgers FJ, Keus RB, et al. Multidimensional assessment of voice characteristics after radiotherapy for early glottic cancer. Laryngoscope 1999;109(2):241–8.

[93] Roh JL, Kim AY, Cho MJ. Xerostomia following radiotherapy of the head and neck affects vocal function. J Clin Oncol 2005;23(13):3016–23.

[94] Fung K, Yoo J, Leeper HA, et al. Vocal function following radiation for non-laryngeal versus laryngeal tumors of the head and neck. Laryngoscope 2001;111(11):1920–4.

[95] Honocodeevar-Boltezar I, Zargi M. Voice quality after radiation therapy for early glottic cancer. Arch Otolaryngol Head Neck Surg 2000;126(9):1097–100.

[96] Cohen SM, Garrett CG, Dupont WD, et al. Voice-related quality of life in T1 glottic cancer: irradiation versus endoscopic excision. Ann Otol Rhinol Laryngol 2006;115(8):581–6.

[97] Fung K, Yoo J, Leeper HA, et al. Effects of head and neck radiation on vocal function. J Otolaryngol 2001;30(3):133–9.

[98] Verdolini K. Guide to vocology. Iowa City (IA): National Center for Voice and Speech; 1998.

[99] Lombard L, Steinhauer K. A novel treatment for hypophonic voice: Twang therapy. J Voice 2007;21:294–9.

[100] Stemple J, Lee L, D'Amico B, et al. Efficacy of vocal function exercises as a method of improving voice production. J Voice 1994;8:271–8.

[101] Casper JK, Murry T. Voice therapy methods in dysphonia. Otolaryngol Clin N Amer 2000;33(5):983–1002.

[102] Roy N, Bless DM, Hiesey D, et al. Manual circumlaryngeal therapy for functional dysphonia: an evaluation of short and long term treatment outcomes. J Voice 1997;11(3):321–31.

[103] Taweechaisupapong S, Pesee M, Aromdee C, et al. Efficacy of pilocarpine lozenge for post-radiation xerostomia in patients with head and neck cancer. Aust Dent J 2006;51(4):333–7.

[104] Aframian DJ, Helcer M, Livni D, et al. Pilocarpine treatment in a mixed cohort of xerostomic patients. Oral Diseases 2007;13(1):88–92.

[105] Dirix P, Nuyts S, Poorten V, et al. Efficacy of the BioXtra dry mouth care system in the treatment of radiotherapy induced xerostomia. Support Care Cancer 2007;15.

[106] LeVeque FG, Montgomery M, Potter D, et al. A multicenter, randomized, double-blind, placebo-controlled, dose-titration study of oral pilocarpine for treatment of radiation-induced xerostomia in head and neck cancer patients. J Clin Oncol 1993;11(6):1124–31.

[107] Chambers MS, Garden AS, Kies MS, et al. Radiation-induced xerostomia in patients with head and neck cancer: pathogenesis, impact on quality of life, and management. Head Neck 2004;26:796–807.

[108] Olsson H, Spak CJ, Axell T. The effect of a chewing gum on salivary secretion, oral mucosal friction, and the feeling of dry mouth in xerostomic patients. Acta Odontol Scand 1991;49:273–9.

[109] Johnstone PA, Peng YP, May BC, et al. Acupuncture for pilocarpine resistant xerostomia following radiotherapy for head and neck malignancies. Int J Radiat Oncol Biol Phys 2001; 50:353–7.

[110] Johnstone PA, Niemtzow RC, Riffenburgh RH. Acupuncture for xerostomia: clinical update. Cancer 2002;94:1151–6.

[111] Verdolini K, Titze IR, Fennell A. Dependence of phonatory effort on hydration level. J Speech Hear Res 1994;37:1001–7.

[112] Forastiere AA, Goepfert H, Maor M, et al. Concurrent chemotherapy and radiotherapy for organ preservation in advanced laryngeal cancer. N Engl J Med 2003;349:2091–8.

[113] Wolf GT, et al. Induction chemotherapy plus radiation compared with surgery plus radiation in patients with advanced laryngeal cancer. N Engl J Med 1991;324:1685–90.

[114] Meleca RJ, Dworkin JP, Kewson DT, et al. Functional outcomes following nonsurgical treatment for advanced-stage laryngeal carcinoma. Laryngoscope 2003;113:720–8.

[115] Orlikoff RF, Kraus DH, Budnick AS, et al. Vocal function following successful chemoradiation treatment for advanced laryngeal cancer: preliminary results. Phonoscope 1999;2:67–77.

[116] Hillman RE, Walsh MJ, Wolf GT, et al. Functional outcomes following treatment for advanced laryngeal cancer. Part I—voice preservation in advanced laryngeal cancer. Part II—laryngectomy rehabilitation. The state of the art in the VA system. Ann Otol Rhinol Laryngol 1998;107:1–27.

[117] Newman LA, Robbins KT, Logemann JA, et al. Swallowing and speech ability after treatment for head and neck cancer with targeted intraarterial versus intravenous chemoradiation. Head Neck 2002;24(1):68–77.

[118] Fung K, Lyden TH, Lee J, et al. Voice and swallowing outcomes of an organ-preservation trial for advanced laryngeal cancer. Int J Radiat Oncol Biol Phys 2005;63(5):1395–9.

[119] Goguen LA, Posner MR, Norris CM, et al. Dysphagia after sequential chemoradiation therapy for advanced head and neck cancer. Otolaryngol Head Neck Surg 2006;134(6): 916–22.

[120] Mowery SE, LoTempio MM, Sadeghi A, et al. Quality of life outcomes in laryngeal and oropharyngeal cancer patients after chemoradiation. Otolaryngol Head Neck Surg 2006; 135(4):565–70.

[121] Gillespie MB, Brodsky MB, Day TA, et al. Swallowing-related quality of life after head and neck cancer treatment. Laryngoscope 2004;114(8):1362–7.

[122] Carrara-de Angelis E, Feher O, Barros AP, et al. Voice and swallowing in patients enrolled in a larynx preservation trial. Arch Otolaryngol Head Neck Surg 2003;129(7): 733–8.

[123] Logemann J, Rademaker A, Pauloski B, et al. Site of disease and treatment protocol as correlates of swallowing function in patients with head and neck cancer treated with chemoradiation. Head Neck 2006;28(1):64–73.

[124] Dworkin JP, Hill SL, Stachler RJ, et al. Swallowing function outcomes following nonsurgical therapy for advanced-stage laryngeal carcinoma. Dysphagia 2006;21(1): 66–74.

[125] Kotz T, Costello R, Li Y, et al. Swallowing dysfunction after chemoradiation for advanced squamous cell carcinoma of the head and neck. Head Neck 2004;26(4):365–72.

[126] Graner DE, Foote RL, Kasperbauer JL, et al. Swallow function in patients before and after intra-arterial chemoradiation. Laryngoscope 2003;113(3):573–9.

[127] Lazarus C. Tongue strength and exercise in healthy individuals and head and neck cancer patients. Semin Speech Lang 2006;27(4):260–7.

[128] Nguyen NP, Frank C, Moltz CC, et al. Impact of dysphagia on quality of life after treatment of head-and-neck cancer. Int J Radiat Oncol Biol Phys 2005;61(3):772–8.

[129] Nguyen NP, Frank C, Moltz CC, et al. Aspiration rate following chemoradiation for head and neck cancer: an underreported occurrence. Radiother Oncol 2006;80(3): 302–6.

[130] Pauloski BR, Rademaker AW, Logemann JA, et al. Pretreatment swallowing function in patients with head and neck cancer. Head Neck 2000;22(5):474–82.

[131] Eisbruch A, Lyden T, Bradford CR, et al. Objective assessment of swallowing dysfunction and aspiration after radiation concurrent with chemotherapy for head-and-neck cancer. Int J Radiat Oncol Biol Phys 2002;53(1):23–8.

[132] Jacobs C, Goffinet DR, Goffinet L, et al. Chemotherapy as a substitute for surgery in the treatment of advanced respectable head and neck cancer: a report from the Northern California Oncology Group. Cancer 1987;60:1178–83.

[133] Jham BC, Freire ARS. Oral complications of radiotherapy in the head and neck. Rev Bras Otorrinolaringol 2006;72(5):704–8.

[134] Jabbari S, Kim HM, Feng M, et al. Matched case-control study of quality of life and xerostomia after intensity-modulated radiotherapy or standard radiotherapy for head-and-neck cancer: initial report. Int J Radiation Oncology Biol Phys 2005;63(3):725–31.

[135] McMillan AS, Pow EH, Kwong DL, et al. Preservation of quality of life after intensity-modulated radiotherapy for early-stage nasopharyngeal carcinoma: results of a prospective longitudinal study. Head Neck 2006;28(8):712–22.

[136] Sasse AD, Clark LG, Sasse EC. Amifostine reduces side effects and improves complete response rate during radiotherapy: results of a meta-analysis. Int J Radiation Oncology Biol Phys 2006;64(3):784–91.

[137] Fife RS, Chase WF, Dore RK, et al. Cevimeline for the treatment of xerostomia in patients with Sjögren syndrome: a randomized trial. Arch Intern Med 2002;162(11):1293–300.

[138] Warde P, Kroll B, O'Sullivan B, et al. A phase II study of Biotene in the treatment of postradiation xerostomia in patients with head and neck cancer. Support Care Cancer 2000;8(3):203–8.

[139] Cohen EG, Deschler DG, Walsh K, et al. Early use of a mechanical stretching device to improve mandibular mobility after composite resection: A pilot study. Arch Phys Med Rehabil 2005;86(7):1416–9.

[140] Sackett DL, Rosenberg WM, Gray JA, et al. Evidence based medicine: what it is and what it isn't. BMJ 1996;312(7023):71–2.

[141] Coyle J, Leslie P. Evidence-based practice: the ethical imperative. Perspectives on swallowing and swallowing disorders 2006; 15(4):1–11.

[142] Logemann JA. Update on clinical trials in dysphagia. Dysphagia 2006;21(2):116–20.

[143] Spencer K. Evidence-based practice: treatment of individuals with dysarthria. Perspectives on neurophysiology and neurogenic speech and language disorders 2006;16(4):13–19.

[144] Perlman AL, Luschei ES, Du Mond CE. Electrical activity from the superior pharyngeal constrictor during reflexive and nonreflexive tasks. J Speech Hear Res 1989;32(4): 749–54.

[145] Clark HM. Neuromuscular treatments for speech and swallowing. Am J Speech Lang Pathol 2003;12(4):400–15.

[146] Stathopoulos E, Duchan JF. History and principles of exercise-based therapy: how they inform our current treatment. Semin Speech Lang 2006;27(4):227–35.

[147] Langmore SE, Terpenning MS, Schork A, et al. Predictors of aspiration pneumonia: how important is dysphagia? Dysphagia 1998;13(2):69–81.

[148] Sapienza C, Wheeler K. Respiratory muscle strength training: functional outcomes versus plasticity. Semin Speech Lang 2006;27(4):236–44.

[149] Kulbersh BD, Rosenthal EL, McGrew BM, et al. Pretreatment, preoperative swallowing exercises may improve dysphagia quality of life. Laryngoscope 2006;116(6):883–6.

[150] Logemann JA, Pauloski BR, Rademaker AW, et al. Super-supraglottic swallow in irradiated head and neck cancer patients. Head Neck 1997;19(6):535–40.

[151] Cichero JAY. Viscosity testing: opening Pandora's box. Perspectives on swallowing and swallowing disorders 2006; 15(1):2–8.

[152] Garcia JM, Chambers E, Matta Z, et al. Viscosity measurements of nectar- and honey-thick liquids: product, liquid, and time comparisons. Dysphagia 2005;20(4):325–35.

[153] Mills RH, Ashford JR. Laboratory assessment battery for dysphagia. Presentation at the Ninth Annual Conference on Head and Neck Rehabilitation: Current Topics in Head and Neck Cancer, Greater Baltimore Medical Center, Baltimore, Maryland, October 27, 2006.

[154] Adachi M, Ishihara K, Abe S, et al. Effect of professional oral health care on the elderly living in nursing homes. Oral Surg Oral Med Oral Pathol Oral Radiol Endod 2002;94(2): 191–5.

[155] Yoneyama T, Yoshida M, Ohrui T, et al. Oral care reduces pneumonia in older patients in nursing homes. J Am Geriatr Soc 2002;50(3):430–3.

ELSEVIER
SAUNDERS

Otolaryngol Clin N Am
41 (2008) 819–823

OTOLARYNGOLOGIC
CLINICS
OF NORTH AMERICA

Index

Note: Page numbers of article titles are in **boldface** type.